DATE DUE

JAN 2 7 2011	
JUN 0 2 2010	
JUN 1 3 2010	
DEC 15 2014	
JUN 09 2015	
DEC 1 8 2015	

D0920198

Tommy Douglas, 1904-1986.

Dave Margoshes

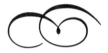

Dave Margoshes is a fiction writer and poet living in Regina. He has published several collections of short stories and two volumes of poetry. His novella, *We Who Seek*, was published in the Fall of 1999 by Black Moss Press. He has won awards for his work, including the 1996 Stephen Leacock Poetry Prize and the 1996 Prairie Fire novella contest. He is the author of a junior high resource book, *Saskatchewan*, part of the Discover Canada series from Grolier. Margoshes worked as a reporter and newspaper editor for over twenty years and also taught journalism for several years. He continues to work occasionally as a freelance journalist; his column appears regularly in *Western Living*, and he writes a regular dispatch from Saskatchewan for *The Vancouver Sun*.

"Margoshes's prose is eloquent and surprising." – *The Globe and Mail*

THE QUEST LIBRARY
is edited by
Rhonda Bailey

The Editorial Board is composed of
Ven Begamudré
Lynne Bowen
Janet Lunn

Editorial correspondence:
Rhonda Bailey, Editorial Director
XYZ Publishing
P.O. Box 250
Lantzville BC
V0R 2H0
E-mail: xyzed@telus.net

In the same collection

Lynne Bowen, *Robert Dunsmuir: Laird of the Mines*.
Betty Keller, *Pauline Johnson: First Aboriginal Voice of Canada*.
John Wilson, *Norman Bethune: A Life of Passionate Conviction*
Rachel Wyatt, *Agnes Macphail: Champion of the Underdog*.

Tommy Douglas

Canadian Cataloguing in Publication Data

Margoshes, Dave, 1941-

    Tommy Douglas : building the new society

    (The Quest Library ; 4)
    Includes bibliographical references and index.

    ISBN 0-9683601-4-9

    1. Douglas, T. C. (Thomas Clement), 1904-1986. 2. Saskatchewan – Politics and government – 1944-1964. 3. Social legislation – Saskatchewan. 4. Prime ministers – Saskatchewan – Biography. 5. Co-operative Commonwealth Federation – Biography. 6. New Democratic Party – Biography I. Title. II. Series.

FC3525.1.D68M37 1999   971.24'03'092   C99-941349-X
F1072.M37 1999

Legal Deposit: Fourth quarter 1999
National Library of Canada
Bibliothèque nationale du Québec

XYZ Publishing acknowledges the support of The Quest Library project by the Canadian Studies Program and the Book Publishing Industry Development Program (BPIDP) of the Department of Canadian Heritage. The opinions expressed do not necessarily reflect the views of the Government of Canada.

The publishers further acknowledge the financial support our publishing program receives from The Canada Council for the Arts, the ministère de la Culture et des Communications du Québec, and the Société de développement des entreprises culturelles.

Chronology: Lynne Bowen
Layout: Édiscript enr.
Cover design: Zirval Design
Cover illustration: Francine Auger

Printed and bound in Canada

XYZ Publishing
1781 Saint Hubert Street
Montreal, Quebec H2L 3Z1
Tel: (514) 525-2170
Fax: (514) 525-7537
E-mail: xyzed@mlink.net

Distributed by: General Distribution Services
325 Humber College Boulevard
Toronto, Ontario M9W 7C3
Tel: (416) 213-1919
Fax: (416) 213-1917
E-mail: customer.service@emailgw.genpub.com

DAVE MARGOSHES

DOUGLAS

Tommy

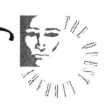

BUILDING THE NEW SOCIETY

XYZ
Publishing

Acknowledgments

There are a number of books, magazine articles, audio-books, and videos about Tommy Douglas available – there are even a few Web sites. Many of these sources are listed in the bibliography at the back. In research-ing this book, I looked at most of the available material, but I found most invaluable *The Making of a Socialist: The Recollections of T.C. Douglas*. Tommy never wrote his autobiography, but this is the next best thing: tran-scriptions of 1958 interviews with the Saskatchewan premier by journalist Chris Higginbotham, placed in the Saskatchewan archives, and edited later by Lewis H. Thomas.

I also made particular use of three other books: two excellent biographies, *Tommy Douglas* by Doris French Shackleton, and *Tommy Douglas: The Road to Jerusalem* by Thomas H. McLeod & Ian McLeod; and a delightful collection of anecdotes, *Touched by Tommy*, edited by Ed and Pemrose Whelan. Thanks very much to Doris French, the McLeods, and the Whelans for permission to use quotes from their books.

I'd also like to acknowledge insights into Tommy's character gleaned from an unpublished doctoral dissertation, *From Preacher to Politician: T.C. Douglas' Transition*, by Jan (John) Oussoren.

Thanks also to Joe Fafard and the Saskatchewan Property Management Corp. for permission to photograph and reproduce the bust of Tommy Douglas by Joe Fafard; and to Macmillan Canada for permission to quote the line in Chapter 4 from W.O. Mitchell's *Who Has Seen the Wind*. (Copyright © W.O. Mitchell, 1947.) Reprinted by permission of Macmillan Canada, an imprint of CDG Books Canada Inc.

Dave Margoshes

Contents

I will not cease from mental fight,
Nor shall my sword sleep in my hand,
Till we have built Jerusalem,
In England's green and pleasant land.
                                                    – William Blake

"Improving people's economic conditions is not
an end in itself, it's a means to an end.... I never
thought a man could save his soul if his belly was
empty or that he could think about things like
beauty and goodness if he had a toothache."
                    – Tommy Douglas in conversation, 1982

"I am conscious of the fact that it is not custom-
ary for ministers to take an active part in the
affairs of the nation; but I also remember that
there was One who went about doing good so
that the common people heard Him gladly. And
I would not be worthy of His name if I did not
take up the sword on behalf of the underpaid
and underprivileged. I therefore dedicate myself
this evening to the service of this constituency...."
                                            – Tommy Douglas
                            in his first nomination speech,
                                              November 4, 1933

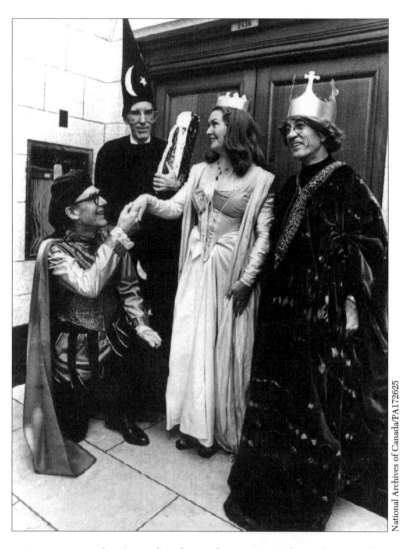

Tommy Douglas (at right) dressed as King Arthur, along with (from left) Conservative Leader Robert Stanfield, Stanley Knowles (as Merlin) and Audrey Schreyer (as Queen Guinevere) in a 1971 Parliamentary Christmas skit, "Chamelot," authored by Stanfield. Tommy was once urged to take up an acting career, "but I never really liked the idea of being an echo of someone else's lines. I wanted to make up my own lines in life."

1

An Immigrant Twice Over

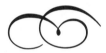

The cold Winnipeg wind whistles around the corner of the house like a freight train bearing down on them, and little Tommy Douglas hunches his thin shoulders, willing the wool of his coat to be thicker and warmer somehow. It's uncomfortable in the sled, the cold and wind, the ice beneath the runners so close to him, every bump shooting through his spine and zeroing-in on his sore knee. But complaint is the farthest thought from his mind. Rather, he's filled with gratitude and wonder at the stoic, silent strength of his two friends who, also uncomplaining, every morning help him into the sled and pull him, across frozen streets, the quarter mile to school.

The pain in his knee is nothing new to Tommy, but just about everything else is. The first years of his young life were spent in the bosom of his father's family in Falkirk, Scotland, where Tommy was the eldest son of an eldest son of an eldest son, all part of a large working-class family of iron moulders. Then, when Tommy was not yet seven, the family packed up their belongings and moved halfway across the world to Winnipeg, on the Canadian frontier. It was 1911 and the world was very different than it is today.

∞

Tommy had been small and sickly almost from birth, and a serious bout with pneumonia when he was six had only made him weaker. Shortly after that, he fell against a stone and hurt the knee of his right leg, an injury that would nag at him for the rest of his life. Osteomyelitis, an infection of the bone, set in and there followed a series of operations on the leg. There was no money for a hospital. Instead, the doctor in his long frock coat and black top hat came to the house. The kitchen was the operating room, with the surgery performed on the table where the family had eaten breakfast shortly before. Young Tommy was sedated with chloroform applied to a gauze mask, his mother, grandmother, and a neighbour woman assisting. The doctor cut an incision in the flesh just above his knee and exposed the infected bone, the femur, so he could scrape it with a knife. No sooner had the doctor left then a suture came out and the wound began to bleed, causing a commotion in the family before it could be stanched.

The Douglas family was already in ferment at this time. Tommy's father, Tom, had fallen prey to the lure of the new world and gone to Canada to check out possibilities, winding up in Winnipeg. As soon as he was settled, the family was to join him. The trip over was delayed by Tommy's injury, but, after two more operations, and months of hobbling around the house and school on crutches, in the early spring of 1911 the leg seemed healed. Tommy, his sister Annie, and their mother, pregnant with another girl, Isobel, set out from Glasgow by ship, seventeen foggy days in the frigid North Atlantic, the trip made all the longer by dangerous sea ice. That was followed by a five-day train trip in the dilapidated old CPR colonist cars, with little kitchens, hot and filled with spicy smells, at the end. The cars were crammed full of immigrant families heading out to the Canadian West – the Great Lone Land – to make their fortunes.

Winnipeg was filling up with families like the Douglases and immigrants from all over Europe speaking so many languages that the city's North End, where most of them gravitated, was like the Tower of Babel. Tom Douglas rented a house on Gladstone Street – it was just a coincidence that the street was named after his own father's hero, William Gladstone, the former British prime minister, and just a coincidence that the neighbourhood was known as Point Douglas. Only one other family on the block the Douglases lived on was from the British Isles, but that made little difference to the kids playing in the street.

Tom Douglas was encouraged by this. He would tell Tommy: "You're playing with the Kravchenko kid. This is marvelous, this is what the world should be like. Sure, I can't understand the family next door, but you kids are growing up together, and you'll work for the same kinds of things, you'll build the same kind of world."

The little house on Gladstone Street (just a block from Winnipeg's notorious red light district on Annabella Street) had an outhouse for a toilet and a pump in the yard for water, but Tommy's mother, a small, lively woman who was forever encouraging Tommy, made a comfortable home there, taking in boarders to help pay the rent. Tommy enrolled at a little schoolhouse on Norquay Street where, while his leg held out, he played some football. He loved the freedom of Winnipeg, where he and his friends could play unfettered along the banks of the Red and Assiniboine rivers, so unlike the confines of Scotland, where most land was private and posted against trespassers.

But it wasn't long before the infection in his knee flared up again, and over the next couple of years he was on crutches most of the time and in and out of the Sick Children's Hospital, undergoing several more operations.

It was during this unhappy period that the neighbour boys made all the difference for Tommy.

All his life, Tommy would vividly remember those boys' acts of kindness that winter when he was ten. He had just come out of hospital and could only walk on crutches. He could get to school in good weather, but when the streets became too clogged with ice and snow, it seemed impossible. It would have been different if his family had a car, but there was only one family in the neighbourhood with such a luxury – later, Tommy remembered that car was "the wonder of the world, and we were allowed to look at it and touch it."

One morning, there was a knock on the door. It was a Polish boy and a Ukrainian boy, fellows Tommy knew from the street and his school, with a sleigh. "They told my mother that they would pull me to school and bring me back each day," Tommy recalled later. There was no request for payment – the boys were motivated just by friendship and kindness. "Those boys speaking broken English, the kind of people that some folks referred to as dagos and foreigners and bohunks, these were the people who came and took an interest in another immigrant boy," he said. "Otherwise, I just wouldn't have got to school."

Tommy Douglas's lifelong hatred for racism, or intolerance of any sort, had already been spoon-fed to him at the knee of both his grandfathers, but it was reinforced that cold day in Winnipeg, and every day of the winter that followed.

He would soon learn another lesson that would stay with him the rest of his life.

Times were tough for his family. His father, used to a good workingman's wage in the iron foundries of Falkirk, could only count on three days' work a week at Winnipeg's Vulcan Iron Works. So whenever Tommy was hospitalized, it put an even greater strain on the Douglas family's pocketbook – in those days, there was no public medical insurance and no employee benefits. In hospital, Tommy was on a ward with other children, and he received the standard medical care – no specialists, certainly no top-notch ones. The doctors did what they could, but eventually they delivered bad news: the leg should come off.

While the family was wrestling with the gut-wrenching decision of whether to let that happen, Tommy happened to come to the attention of Dr. R.H. Smith, a well-known orthopedic surgeon who was leading a group of medical students through Tommy's ward.

Dr. Smith paused at the foot of Tommy's bed, exchanged a few pleasantries with the boy, who was homesick and in pain but cheerful nonetheless, and flipped through his chart. He read of one failed medical procedure and operation after another, and the awful prognosis. The case interested him. When Tommy's parents came for a visit later, the surgeon had a proposition for them: he'd take over and try a tricky form of surgery that just might save Tommy's leg, although it would probably leave the knee permanently stiffened. All they had to do was allow him to use the operation as a teaching exercise, with the students watching. How could they refuse?

"As a result of several operations, he saved my leg," Tommy said later.

In fact, the operation was even more successful than anyone imagined. As an adult, Tommy Douglas liked to tell the story of how, after the knee had healed, the great surgeon and his students gathered around the young patient to remove the bandages and inspect the handiwork. Dr. Smith poked and prodded and pronounced himself satisfied – up to a point. "It's too bad he cannot bend his knee," he told the suitably impressed students.

"But Doctor, I can bend it," the young patient exclaimed. And he did!

Years later, after another injury, the old bad knee would come back to plague him. But so successful was Dr. Smith's handiwork that for the next thirty years, Tommy Douglas was able to hike, bike, kick soccer balls, box, and keep up with the strenuous rigours of political campaigning.

Tommy had been very lucky. "When I thought about it," he recalled, "I realized that the same kind of service I got by a stroke of luck should have been available to every child in that ward, and not just to a case that looked like a good specimen for exhibition to medical students."

He always felt a debt of gratitude to the doctor who came to his rescue, "but it left me with this feeling that if I hadn't been so fortunate as to have this doctor offer me his services gratis, I would probably have lost my leg. I felt that no boy should have to depend either for his leg or his life upon the ability of his parents to raise enough money to bring a first-class surgeon to his bedside. And I think it was out of this experience, not at the moment consciously, but through the years, I came to believe that health services ought not to have a price-tag on them, and that people should be able to get whatever health services they required irrespective of their individual capacity to pay."

And so it was that the germ that developed into the national health care program was planted in the mind of the boy who would grow up to become the premier of Saskatchewan and to be known across Canada as the "father of medicare."

Thomas Clement Douglas was born in Falkirk, Scotland, on October 20, 1904, the first of three children of Tom Douglas, a recently returned veteran of the Boer War, and Anne Clement, daughter of Highlanders who had migrated to Glasgow. The birth was an auspicious one that brought about a reconciliation between Tom and his own father, also named Thomas, a stern, demanding disciplinarian who was noted in the community as a fiery orator.

The elder Thomas was a lifelong Liberal who took pride in having once introduced William Gladstone at a political rally. His son came home from South Africa sickened by the horrors and injustices of war and, shortly after, announced that he had switched allegiances to the relatively new Labour Party, the socialists. The father threw the son out of his house and for over a year the two didn't speak.

But after little Tommy's birth, the proud grandfather couldn't stay away long. One day there was a knock at the door, and there stood the elder Thomas Douglas, "come to see the boy."

Over the next few years, each of the old man's other seven sons "went Labour," and eventually he too made the switch, so Tommy Douglas, who would become the head of the first socialist government in North America in 1944, came by his politics honestly.

The town of Falkirk, about midway between Glasgow and Edinburgh, lies close to the site of a decisive battle in 1297 between British troops and Scottish forces led by William Wallace. The great iron works that was established there, fuelled by coal from nearby mines, made cannons for Wellington during the

Napoleonic Wars. The men of the Douglas clan had worked at the iron works for several generations. It was a large and loving family, and little Tommy, as the first grandson and because he was always a bit sickly, was particularly loved. Although his father was a working man, he made a comfortable living by Falkirk standards, and Tommy enjoyed a happy childhood, except for his health problems.

The Douglas clan lived in two stone houses owned by Grandfather Douglas at the foot of a brae, the Scottish word for hill. At the time of Tommy's birth, the houses still had thatched roofs, though later the thatch was replaced with slate, and they were heated by fireplaces. There was a lot of reading done in those houses and a lot of arguing, about politics, religion, philosophy. It was a stimulating environment for a bright, observant boy like Tommy, a daydreamer who chafed at the limits placed on him by his poor health.

His grandfather Douglas had the large callused hands and broad shoulders of an ironworker, but he was a Sunday painter. In addition to introducing Gladstone, he had painted a portrait of the great man. And, most significantly for his young grandson, he was an amateur orator with a wide reputation – Tommy remembered him as "one of the finest speakers I ever heard"– and had committed to memory hundreds of verses of Robert Burns, Scotland's beloved national poet. Tommy's earliest memories were of sitting on the old man's knee by the fireside as he recited lines from "Tam o' Shanter" and other famous Burns poems.

Young Tommy absorbed Scottish history and the nationalism, egalitarianism, and religious fervour of

Burns. A boyhood hero was Robert the Bruce, a thirteenth century Scottish king who battled the British. Years later, after losing his first election, Tommy would remind his supports that Robert only won a decisive victory after having first been beaten six times.

Tommy's dad was a big, burly man who, nevertheless, liked to grow roses in his small Falkirk garden. He'd stopped going to church after a falling out with the minister. He associated the Presbyterians with the rich and Liberals; that party, he said, was made up of "conniving hypocrites" and was no friend to working people, a view Tommy adopted himself. Tom Douglas had left school at thirteen to begin work and, just as he had been the first in his family to change politics, for his son he aspired to something different from an iron moulder's life. He wanted an education for the boy, and freedom from the restrictions of Great Britain's rigid class system. He began to think about life in "the colonies."

The Douglases hadn't been in Canada for more than three years before the First World War broke out and Tom, as a British reservist, was called back to duty, joining an ambulance unit. The rest of the family, rather than stay in Canada without a breadwinner, sailed back to Scotland on the *Pretoria*, travelling without lights through U-boat-infested waters – a thrilling trip for a ten-year-old boy. They took up residence in Glasgow with Annie Douglas's parents, the Clements.

Tommy's grandfather Andrew Clement was a teamster who drove a delivery wagon for a co-operative market and was a great supporter of the co-op movement that, years later, the grandson would champion in Saskatchewan.

Tommy's future as an amateur boxer began to make itself evident when he began school.

Like many boys around the world, he had to contend with bullies. On his first day, he set off for the Scotland Street School decked out in gartered knickers and a little porkpie hat, regular attire for Canadian schoolboys of the day. As he passed a corner that was the territory of a tough gang, he was met with gales of laughter. "Hey, Canuck," the boys yelled, and one of them knocked off his hat. Tommy was small but his years in an out of hospital had made him somewhat immune to pain – and pugnacious as hell. When a big boy called Geordie Sinclair told him to jump, Tommy refused.

"Do it or I'll belt you," Geordie said, but Tommy stood his ground – and got a bloody nose.

Although Tommy punched Geordie right back, in the tussle that followed he was no match for the bigger boy.

Just the same, the next day, after school, Tommy went looking for Geordie and his chums. Taking a deep breath, he issued a challenge: "If you haven't had enough, I'll give you some more. Are you ready?"

Sometimes bluff works. And grit.

Instead of kicking the tar out of Tommy, or bursting into laughter, Geordie Sinclair was impressed. "You've had enough, Canuck," he declared.

Tommy wasn't bothered anymore, and he and Geordie became pals.

⚭

His leg healthy and pain free, Tommy was able to fully enjoy his childhood for the first time. Though he was no great shakes at his studies, after graduating from elementary school he enrolled in a private high school academy. He became close to his grandfather and spent many hours helping him on his rounds and caring for his horses. In his spare time, Tommy would often go to church, not because he was particularly religious, but to listen in fascination to the preachers. And he and a pal, Tom Campbell, loved nothing better than a Sunday afternoon jaunt to Glasgow Green, where they would listen to a succession of socialists and other soapbox speakers railing against the establishment.

But he was an obedient boy himself. "I didn't rebel because there was nobody to rebel against," he recalled.

With his dad away in the war, money was tight and Tommy took a series of part-time jobs to pay his way at school. What he really wanted to do was go to sea as a sailor, but he was too young. One of his best jobs was as a soap boy in a barbershop, working evenings and all day Saturday, rubbing soap into the bristly whiskers of men waiting for a shave, for which he earned six shillings a week plus tips. He was a likable boy and did well with the tips – at Christmas, he made an extra two pounds, a lot of money for a thirteen-year-old.

The next summer, he got a job in a cork factory, for thirty shillings a week. The owner took a liking to Tommy, and soon he was promoted to office work, at three pounds a week, more than his father had ever earned in the iron works! Tommy was getting on so well at the factory that he didn't bother going back to school in the fall, which made his father blow his top when he came home on leave.

But the war was almost over, and Canada was calling to the family again. On New Year's Day 1919, with Tommy just having turned fourteen, the family set sail once more. This time, they would be in Canada for good.

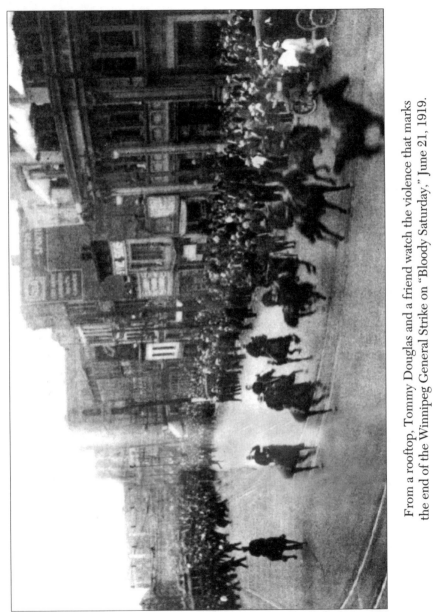

From a rooftop, Tommy Douglas and a friend watch the violence that marks the end of the Winnipeg General Strike on "Bloody Saturday," June 21, 1919.

2

Boxing Rings and Grease Paint

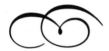

June 21, 1919 – "Bloody Saturday." A front page photo in the paper this evening shows vividly a climactic moment in the violence that marks the end of the Winnipeg General Strike.

It's a panoramic view of Main Street in the throes of a riot. The famous streetcar the strikers overturned and set ablaze is over there, and there, at the left, lies the body of a man gunned down by police. Crowds mill in the background and on the sides.

The photo is dominated by a troop of uniformed RCMP officers, charging down the street on their horses and brandishing clubs.

And over there, slightly above the centre, you can just make out the shapes of two figures on a rooftop, watching the horrific scene, never to be forgotten, unfold before them.

The two are fourteen-year-old Tommy Douglas and a friend.

"We were too stupid to be scared up there," Tommy remembered. "We were just excited by it all."

∞

Tommy and his mother and two sisters had arrived back in Winnipeg early in the year and rented a house on Gordon Street, not far from where they'd lived a few years earlier. Tom Douglas, still not mustered out of the army, would follow in a few months. Anne Douglas got a job at the Singer sewing machine factory. Tommy had every intention of honouring his father's wishes and returning to school, but, for the moment, money was tight, and he too went to work.

So it was that he and another boy, Mark Talnicoff – who would later marry Tommy's sister Annie – were delivering copies of a newspaper in the Market Square near city hall on that Saturday afternoon when they heard the commotion. The two boys shimmied up a pole and made it to the roof of a two-story building on Main Street near the corner of Williams Street, right in the heart of the tumult, just as shots started to ring out. Police fired in the air at first, and several bullets whizzed by the boys' heads. They ducked, scared and exhilarated, but they didn't turn and run.

From their vantage point, they could see everything: the streetcar tipped over, the fighting, the charge of the Mounties, the shootings and clubbings that left two men dead and many others wounded. It was the culmination of the city's – and country's – first ever general strike, then in its thirty-eighth day, and would break the strike's back. Scores of strike leaders were rounded up over the next few days, including the Douglas family's pastor, James Woodsworth, and several of them were tried and sent to prison.

Tommy remembered the scene this way: "We saw the mounted police and the men who had been taken in as sort of vigilantes riding from North Main straight down toward the corner of Portage and Main, then re-forming on Portage Avenue and coming back down again, riding the strikers down and breaking up the meetings, breaking up their parade.

"There was quite a good deal of shooting. Most of the mounted policemen were shooting into the air, but some of them shot into the crowd."

Although Tommy wasn't directly involved in the strike, he retained vivid memories of the fist-waving speeches given by strike leaders like Fred Dixon, John Queen, and the gaunt, bearded Woodsworth, who had become a sort of role model for the boy.

Woodsworth, usually known by his initials, J.S., was a Methodist minister and head of the All People's Mission, a combination social centre and school where Anne Douglas was a volunteer and Tommy often used the library and sports facilities. He was a soft-spoken man who suddenly turned into a lion when he stepped on a soapbox. A strong advocate of the concept of "practical Christianity," or the social gospel, "in the part of society that we moved in, he was a little god," Tommy said. He would be elected to Parliament as a

Labour candidate in two years and would become a colleague of Tommy's fifteen years later. Now, it was shocking news to hear that Woodsworth had been arrested.

"It's an awful disgrace when your minister goes to jail," Tommy said.

The Winnipeg strike left an indelible impression on Tommy Douglas, who became increasingly interested in politics and began to work in local campaigns, handing out leaflets and doing other small chores. It wasn't just the jailing of Woodsworth and the violence he witnessed on Bloody Saturday that effected him.

"Not until after the Estevan riot (which Tommy also witnessed, a dozen years later) and later the Regina riot (in 1934) did I realize that this was all part of a pattern," he would recall. "Whenever the powers that be can't get what they want, they're always prepared to resort to violence or any kind of hooliganism to break the back of organized opposition."

Three years later, another fight. The scene is an old arena on Main Street across from the Union Station by the Fort Garry Hotel. A Saturday night in spring, and there's a big crowd. The smells of beer and sweat are in the air, and there's an all-but-palpable sense of excitement. The main event is about to begin, and this time, Tommy isn't watching – he's in the thick of it.

In the sixth and final round of their championship fight, defending champ Cecil Matthews and the challenger, seventeen-year-old Tommy Douglas, are tied on

points. Tommy is small and, by his own admission, "not
a particularly outstanding boxer. I was too short in the
arm to be a good boxer, but I was fast on my feet and
could hit fairly hard."

But this day in 1922, Tommy gets a lucky break.
With the clock ticking down, Matthews gets careless.
He tries to come in fast and go under Tommy's guard;
in the process, he drops his own guard and leaves himself wide open. Wham! Tommy connects. It's not a
knockout but it's enough to win the round for Tommy,
and the fight, and with it the amateur lightweight
championship of Manitoba.

∞

You'd think a boy's parents would be proud of this kind
of achievement. Not Tommy's – they were disgusted.
Anne Douglas's religious scruples were too strict to see
boxing as anything less than the devil's work, and Tom
had seen enough violence in two wars to last a lifetime. On the trail to the championship, their son had
collected a broken nose, a couple of lost teeth, a
strained hand, and a sprained thumb. Now they
looked him over, his face red and puffy, his hand
throbbing with pain, and they shook their heads sadly.
"It serves you right," Tom declared. "If you're fool
enough to get into this sort of thing, don't ask for any
sympathy."

Nor did Tommy get any.

Tommy had begun boxing when he was fifteen
and weighed in at 135 pounds (61 kg). He used to go
to the gym operated by the One Big Union, a labour

organization that had sprung up during the General Strike, and was attracted by the lure of the ring. After all those years tied to a crutch, Tommy was now remarkably fast on his feet. He found himself cast as a sparring partner for Lloyd Peppen, who became Canadian lightweight champion, and Charlie Balongey, who went on to be a heavyweight champ. He continued to fight through his teenage years, and his boxing culminated in the championship, which he successfully defended the following year, when he was eighteen.

Tommy Douglas the boxer! That was something the doctors who worked on the skinny boy's infected leg a few years earlier would never have expected. But the Tommy Douglas who returned to Winnipeg in 1919 was a far different boy than the one who had left it four years earlier.

Until Tom Douglas rejoined them that spring, Tommy assumed many of the responsibilities in the family, and the fourteen-year-old boy grew up in a hurry. Indeed, from the time Tommy returned to Canada, as the Bible says, he pretty much put aside childish things and began to speak like a man.

"I was the man of the family," he'd recall, "and had to look after things: see that the storm windows were put up, and that my sisters would start school – I went with them and got them placed – and this sort of thing. And this isn't bad for a boy."

Even after his father came home, Tommy continued to play more of an adult's role than that of a boy.

Tom Douglas was weakened, both physically, from exposure to gas in the trenches, and emotionally. For his service to king and country, he was awarded a bonus, which the family used as a down payment for a house on McPhail Street, near the Elmwood Cemetery. He also received a military pension of about twelve dollars a month, not nearly enough to live on, and he soon returned to the iron works. It was dangerous work and twice Tom narrowly escaped serious injury when he was splashed with molten metal. For the rest of his life, he would be the victim of frequent bouts of depression, and whatever dreams of a better life he had that had brought him to Canada would have to be played out in his children.

But it would take a while. Times were tough for the Douglases in the twenties, and even Annie and Isobel went to work, as sales clerks, after finishing grade school. As for Tommy, he wanted to go back to school but thought his father "was living in a dream world" if he imagined the family could afford such a luxury.

Tommy's first job was as a messenger boy for a drug store at the corner of Higgins and Main, near the Royal Alex Hotel, and he earned six dollars a week. But he was an ambitious boy and, always on the lookout for better opportunities, soon answered an ad from the Richardson Press, which produced a variety of publications, including the *Grain Trade News*.

He went to the print shop and told the foreman he wanted a job. The man looked Tommy over and tried him out on a few things, and then said, "I'll teach you all I know, and you still won't know anything."

As it turned out, Tommy would work as an apprentice printer for five years, thoughts of school and an education put aside. He started out as what was known as a printer's devil, doing odd, dirty jobs in the always-dirty print shop. He broke lead type out of its wooden forms, melted it down for reuse, and scrubbed the ever-present ink off machines, walls, and furniture with gasoline. Soon he moved on to setting type, working full time Monday through Friday and half a day Saturday. By the time he was sixteen, Tommy was the youngest Linotype operator in Canada, earning full journeyman's wages, forty-five dollars a week, even though he was still an apprentice.

Aside from work, his life was busy.

Two nights, he took printing classes; the rest of the week, he was active in church groups at the nearby Beulah Baptist Church and in Boy Scouts and the Order of DeMolay, a youth wing of the Masons, which his father had joined. As a Scout, Tommy quickly rose to troop leader, patrol leader, cubmaster and, eventually, scoutmaster. He loved working with kids younger than he was, a fact that would play a large part in his later decision to become a minister.

He also joined the militia, the 79th Cameron Highlanders, earning a small stipend for playing the clarinet in the band and wearing kilts on parade.

Tommy was active in sports, in addition to the boxing, primarily through the Scouts. His was a cycling troop – all the boys in his Elmwood neighbourhood had jobs and owned their own bicycles. "We painted them red with grey trimmings," he remembered, "and on the weekends, we'd put packs on our backs and go out on the open road by East St. Paul (a Winnipeg suburb) and camp out. We'd go out on Saturday afternoon, and come back Sunday night or early Monday morning." On these trips, their backpacks would be stuffed with baseballs and gloves, soccer balls and other sports equipment.

As for the boxing, he not only embraced it himself, but encouraged the boys in his Scout troop to give it a try. "That doesn't mean I'd like any boy to get into professional boxing," he said. "But you don't avoid fights by never fighting. I think you avoid fights if somebody knows that you're willing to fight."

More significantly for his future life, he was a voracious reader, tackling books on politics and religion as well as the English novels, like the romances of Sir Walter Scott, he devoured; and the world of amateur theatre opened up for him. Those recitations of Robbie Burns by his grandfather Douglas had made a lasting impression, and Tommy, who had inherited his grandfather's prodigious memory, began performing monologues, which were very popular at the time. This was in the days before television or even radio, and people went in for homemade entertainment. He took lessons with a famous Winnipeg elocutionist, Jean Campbell, who herself was a student of Jean Alexander, a nationally famous speaker and writer. Tommy became a hit attraction at Burns dinners – an annual occurrence on the great poet's birthday – and at Masonic and other functions, where he would recite poems by Burns, Kipling, and Pauline Johnson, the Canadian Indian woman who was then all the rage. Sometimes the Scouts would organize concerts, with Tommy as one of the attractions, and sell tickets for a quarter.

Whatever fear of audiences Tommy may have had quickly evaporated. "It was excellent training for a life in politics," he remembered, although at this point a life in politics was the farthest thing from his mind.

His active life made him "a bit of an oddity in the print shop," he remembered. "I was always good friends with everyone, but I didn't join the lads in the evenings. I didn't go to the drinking parties and didn't play poker, as most printers do. And at noon hour, whenever there was a poker game, I was usually memorizing a recitation for the evening or getting a little talk ready." But, he added with a straight face, "I was provincial lightweight champion, and so they didn't kid me too much."

Two men were strong influences on Tommy during this period of his boyhood.

Through the DeMolays, he became close to W.J. Major and Dr. "Dad" Howden, who were sort of big brothers with the group.

Major, a lawyer who would later become attorney general of Manitoba and a Queen's Bench judge, was largely responsible for persuading Tommy to return to school. He pointed out that the young man seemed to have talent aplenty, but without formal schooling, his potential was severely limited.

His other mentor, Howden, owned the Winnipeg Theatre and was a part owner in the Walker Theatre, a major stop in the vaudeville circuit, and Tommy and other boys would often attend performances with him. Gradually, Tommy began to get small roles, playing a butler or making good use of his Scottish accent.

Howden was so impressed he offered to pay Tommy's way if he wanted to quit his job and take up dramatic training. But Tommy never took the stage that seriously.

"The experience gave me a feel for grease paint," he said, "but I never really liked the idea of being an echo of someone else's lines. I wanted to make up my own lines in life."

His life on the stage led to one personally memorable moment, though.

As an understudy for one of the major roles at a play to be performed at a Masonic convention, Tommy stepped in without blinking an eye when the leading man had to drop out. He got a standing ovation from the five thousand Masons who saw him. Tommy would never forget what happened later that evening.

His father had been in the audience and was justifiably proud. But Tom Douglas was a reticent man who was sparing of praise, especially for his son.

"Let's walk," he said, as the two of them emerged from the old Board of Trade Building downtown. They walked in silence up Main Street and then along Henderson Road and through their old Point Douglas neighborhood, then across the Disraeli Bridge over the Red River and into Elmwood to the small old house at 132 McPhail Street.

"I knew from that he'd been deeply moved by the performance," Tommy recalled. "We never exchanged a word all the way home, but, as we were going up the front step, he tapped me on the shoulder and said, 'You did no bad.' That was as close as he ever came to giving me a word of praise. He might tell my mother that he was pleased, but he found it very difficult to tell me."

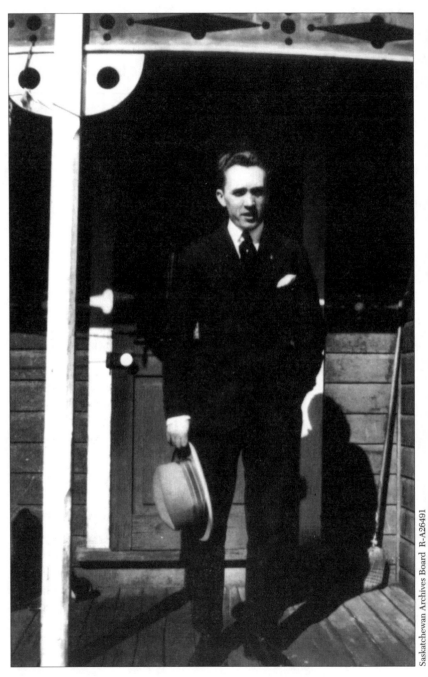

As a supply preacher to rural congregations, Douglas is so popular that sixteen-year-old Irma Dempsey comes to hear him and falls in love.

3

A Commitment to the Church

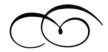

A Sunday morning in spring, 1922, the Canadian National Railway station at Stonewall, Manitoba, a short ride north of Winnipeg.

A young man dressed in his best suit steps tentatively out of a coach and onto the crowded platform. He's nineteen but he's small, slender, baby-faced, and looks more like fourteen.

The whole congregation of the Stonewall Baptist Church, about forty people, are milling about on the platform, looking for the man sent up from Winnipeg to be their preacher for the day. Nobody takes any notice of the shy young man, on his first assignment as a lay preacher.

Since no one pays any attention to him, he goes up to a boy who is leaning against his bicycle. "Can you tell me how to get to the Baptist church?"

The boy looks at the young man in surprise. "What do you want at the Baptist church?" he asks suspiciously.

"I'm supposed to be taking the service this morning," the young man answers.

"Are you the new preacher?"

"Yes, I am."

Then, in a loud voice, the boy calls out: "Ma, this kid says he's the new preacher!"

All eyes turn to Tommy Douglas and, he would recall later, "the disappointment in their faces was very noticeable."

Just the same, his service is a success – and he's invited back.

∞

Tommy Douglas seems to have been born to the preacher's trade, just as he was born to the life of a politician.

Both his grandfathers had been religious men. Old Thomas Douglas was a devout follower of Scotland's establishment Presbyterian Church who, despite his love of Burns and Scotch whisky, frowned on singing and dancing, particularly on the Sabbath. Andrew Clement had, as a young man, been a drunkard who was "saved" by the ultra-conservative Christian Brethren. A sober, quiet man at the time Tommy knew him, he had become a lay Baptist preacher who often would stop to deliver sermons as he made his rounds as a delivery man.

Anne Douglas was also quite religious and, in Winnipeg, steered her family to the Baptist Church, always harbouring the hope that her son would be attracted to the ministry. The whole family, with the exception of Tom Douglas, who had little use for religion, became active in the neighbourhood Beulah Baptist Church.

When he was studying to be a preacher, Tommy remembered a time when the straitlaced minister of the Beulah church came to call on the Douglases around supper time. Tom arrived home from work shortly afterwards and, as was his custom, tramped into the kitchen in his dirty pants and boots, the smell of molten metal still clinging to him.

"I'm going to have a bottle of beer," he told their guest. "Would you like one?"

The minister declined. Anne and the children were mortified by this behaviour, but later Tommy came both to value that forthrightness in his father and to learn a lesson about the clergy. If he was to be a minister, he decided, it would be one who would welcome a glass of beer at a parishioner's home, who would accept his parishioners as he found them and would strive to be one with them.

Tommy's first taste of a preacher's life came when he was fifteen or sixteen and was appointed chaplain of his DeMolay chapter. His role was to give a prayer at the start of meetings. He usually just read the words from a book, but one night, after several children had been injured in a fire in the city, he was pressed into tailoring a special prayer, which he successfully improvised.

Beulah was a conservative church, with the emphasis on salvation and the afterlife, on doing good works to insure getting into Heaven, not for their own sake. But Tommy, with J.S. Woodsworth as a role model, was developing decidedly more liberal religious views. He and his good friend Mark Talnicoff (later changed to Talney), a fellow Scout leader, would spend hours discussing politics and religion, and their talks focused on the increasingly intriguing notion of the social gospel, "the application of the gospel to social conditions," as Tommy later described it. They saw themselves as rebels. The germ of the idea to become a preacher was planted in Tommy's head, but not because he had "a call." Rather, he and Mark saw the church as a way of working for social change.

One chilly night, walking home from church, the two boys decided that the ministry was for them, and they started thinking about Brandon College, a combination liberal arts and Bible school run by the Baptist Church. Brandon College was a hotbed of liberal ideas and was just a couple of hours' train ride west of Winnipeg.

As it turned out, it would be another year or so before either of them actually made it to college. Tommy used that year to read as much as he could, to take on practice preaching assignments like the one at Stonewall and other nearby country churches, and to set a little money aside.

Tommy made good money as a printer, more than his father, but most of it went to help pay off the mortgage on the family home. For a year, he made special efforts to save money toward college, although when he did arrive at Brandon, in the fall of 1924, just a few weeks before his twentieth birthday, he had only ninety dollars in his pocket.

As it is with many students, money was always an issue for Tommy during his entire six years at Brandon: three years making up for his missed high school, and three as a theology student, or "theolog." To make ends meet, he made himself available as a public speaker and performer at concerts and dances, as he had in Winnipeg, doing monologues and recitations at five dollars a performance. That first fall in Brandon, he was the star of the fowl-supper circuit for miles around the city.

In his first couple of years at college, Tommy took on other odd jobs to make a few dollars, waiting on tables and acting as late-night doorman at the dormitory. Students who came in after the doors were locked had to ring a bell and were fined a quarter. As Tommy remembered it: "You kept the twenty-five cents for getting up and opening the door. Any fellow who wakes you up at one o'clock in the morning deserves to pay two bits."

More importantly, he joined other students and became an active "supply" preacher, working all through his college years – even while he was still technically in high school – on weekends and summers at neighbouring rural churches, too small to afford a full-time preacher.

In fact, even before he'd arrived at Brandon, he had his first paying assignment: on his way to the college, he was to get off the train at the small town of Austin, about midway between Portage la Prairie and Brandon, and do a quick job, winding things up at a church that was being disbanded.

"The church had been going to pieces," he told an interviewer years later. "They'd had a row and half the congregation had become British Israelites. And so I was to go and have this service, close them off formally, and bury the dead." He thought it was a shame, though, that differences about biblical interpretation should deprive the youngsters of the community of religious education. "At twenty years of age, you're brash and ready to hand out advice to people three times your age with complete equanimity. So I proceeded to preach a sermon saying it was disgraceful that they were closing this church."

Afterwards, the congregation met and the deacon came sheepishly to Tommy "and admitted they had been a little foolish." If he would agree to come every Sunday, they'd try to make a go of their church for another year.

Brandon College officials took a dim view of a first-year student having such a heavy load, but they agreed to allow him to preach every other Sunday, with his friend Mark Talney sharing the position, at fifteen dollars for each Sunday.

Tommy also spent two summers in Austin. "The first summer, I got around to all the farms on a bicycle," he remembered. "The next year they got me an old Ford car; it took me halfway and I pushed it the rest."

After two years, Tommy was assigned to a Presbyterian church in Carberry, just a short train ride east of Brandon. Although the Knox Church wasn't Baptist, it was desperate for a minister and appealed to the college. Ecumenicalism worked to Tommy's advantage in another way at Carberry as well. His reputation as a preacher attracted the attentions of a pretty girl named Irma Dempsey, a petite, brown-haired Methodist with shining eyes who came to hear him one Sunday and quickly changed churches. It was the start of a romance that would blossom into marriage.

Tommy was in Carberry for two years, then was reassigned to Baptist churches in the Shoal Lake and Strathclair area, a couple of hours northwest of Brandon. He would take a Saturday afternoon train to Minnedosa, where he'd change to a train to Strathclair. He'd spend the night with an elderly farm family named Kippen, two brothers and two sisters who would make sure to get him to the church on time – Shoal Lake in the afternoon, Strathclair in the evening – by old Model T Ford in good weather, a team and cutter in the winter.

Finally, in his last year at Brandon, Tommy was sent for a tryout to Weyburn, Saskatchewan, where the Calvary Baptist Church was looking for a permanent minister.

Tommy was extremely popular as a student minister, especially among children. He organized drama and sports clubs, showed them the manly art of boxing, and regaled them with tales of big-city Winnipeg. At Sunday school, he always had stories and jokes, and one of his favourites involved a bit of sleight of hand. He would flash a shining red heart, cut out of construction paper, and caution the children what might happen if they lied, stole, or were disrespectful to their parents. He would say some magic words and – presto! – the red heart would be replaced with a coal black one.

On September 29, 1929, he wrote a message in the autograph book of a young parishioner in Shoal Lake:

Dear Wilma,
If instead of giving gems or flowers, we could drop a beautiful thought into the heart of a friend, that would be giving as the angels give.
T.C. Douglas.

∞

Demanding as this practice preaching was, Tommy also was taking a full load at Brandon. He excelled in his studies, which included Greek and Hebrew, and he won top marks in the latter, in a class that included several Jews studying to be rabbis. He was head of his class for the first three years. Then he met his match in the form of Stanley Knowles, another printer newly arrived at the college. The careers of Knowles and Douglas would have many parallels – both became Baptist ministers and both became distinguished left-wing politicians, with Knowles reigning as "the dean of Parliament" until his retirement in 1984. For the moment, though, they were the friendliest of rivals, dividing academic honours between them, though Knowles scored more gold medals in their graduation year.

"I tried to take the gold medals but they made me put them back," Tommy quipped.

To which Knowles retorted: "Tommy was smarter, but I was better at writing exams."

Brandon College was an affiliate of McMaster University in Windsor, Ontario, another Baptist-founded school. At the time, the Baptist Church was polarized by radical and fundamental views on a wide range of theological issues, and many Baptists would have been scandalized to learn what was taught in the hallowed halls at Brandon that they helped to support. The notorious Scopes "monkey" trial, which had pitted the theory of Darwinism against religious fundamentalism in the United States, had played itself out only a couple of years before Tommy enrolled at Brandon, and many Baptists were on the fundamentalist side. But at the college, liberal ideas were given full rein (ironically, Brandon College was noted for its geology program, which taught a theory of an earth millions of years old that was diametrically opposed to the biblical view), and a charge of heresy had been levied against several Brandon professors. Tommy sarcastically described the position of the fundamentalists this way: "I want complete freedom of thought unless your point of view is different from mine, in which case you'll believe what I believe."

The Brandon faculty was cleared, but the controversy continued, a cloud hanging over the college until, in 1938, the Baptists would cut their ties. In the meantime, though, the idea of the social gospel held sway at Brandon College, the idea that the church should be as concerned with the welfare of the human body as that of the soul, that the church should be an instrument for change and justice. Tommy thrived in this atmosphere of openness and intellectual rigour. His views on Christianity, already influenced by left-wing political thought, became even more liberal, and he developed a sense of biblical truth as a metaphor for human behaviour not as it necessarily is but as it should be. And the way he articulated his thoughts was increasingly popular, even among the conservative, rural congregations he preached to on Sundays all through his school days.

Tommy explained his approach to preaching this way: "You start with a text. But the Bible is like a bull fiddle, you can play almost any tune you want on it. My background, being interested in social and economic questions, naturally inclined me to preaching the idea that religion in essence was entering into a new relationship with God and into a new relationship with the universe. And into a new relationship with your fellow man. And that if Christianity meant anything, it meant building the brotherhood of man.

"And that meant a helpful relationship between man and man, building a society and building institutions that would uplift mankind, and particularly those that were the least fortunate. This was pretty well the message I was trying to get across."

∞

Tommy also threw himself wholeheartedly into other aspects of college life. He was a champion debater, and a team he led beat all comers, including a prestigious Oxford University team from England that was touring Canada. He also took part in dramatics, the student newspaper, and student government, serving as "senior stick" – president of the student body – in his last year.

He also developed a reputation on campus as a practical joker who, despite his achievements, didn't take himself too seriously.

And he still found time for romance.

In Carberry, Tommy would often visit Irma Dempsey at her parents' farm, where her father was a horse dealer. Tommy knew something about horses from his boyhood years in Glasgow when he would accompany his grandfather Clement on his delivery rounds and help him care for his horses and rig. And a good thing, too. "If I hadn't been able to talk to Irma's dad about horses," Tommy said, "I doubt that he would have ever let me marry his daughter."

After finishing high school, Irma, who played piano, moved to Brandon to study music at the college, where their relationship became even more serious.

"They used to warn the girls at college to stay away from the theologs," Tommy remembered, "or they'd end up in a drafty manse somewhere, getting their clothes out of a missionary box."

Irma wasn't dissuaded. They were married in the summer of 1930, shortly after Tommy's graduation and ordination. Mark Talney, already ordained, married them; Stanley Knowles was best man. Tommy was not quite twenty-six and Irma was barely nineteen; together, they were on their way to Saskatchewan.

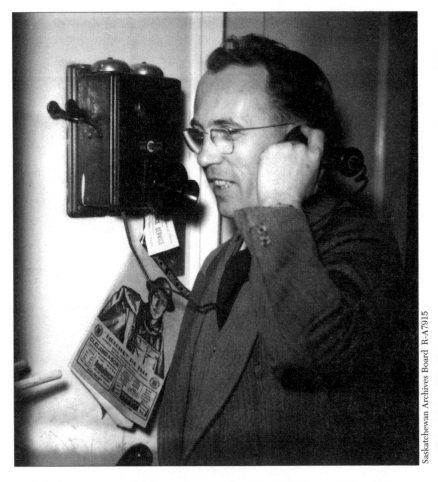

While the minister of Calvary Baptist Church in Weyburn, Saskatchewan, Douglas organizes the unemployed. "We believe that any society, most of all a Christian society, is measured by what it does for the aged, for the sick, the orphans and the less fortunate who live in our midst."

4

Dustbowl Preacher

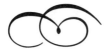

Summer, 1931, Chicago. The notorious "hobo jungle," a massive shantytown sprung up practically overnight along the railroad tracks that crisscross the city.

The Depression is less than two years old, but already millions of men are out of work.

Jobless, homeless men lounge in small groups around open fires, talking quietly. There's no drinking, but the sense of hopelessness that wafts off the shoulders of the men like cold fog gives a sense of menace to the scene. It's late, past midnight. A sliver of moon blinks on and off like neon as clouds speed across the navy blue sky.

A group of young men, dressed in pleated slacks and loafers, carrying notebooks, move warily, nervously, through the clusters of men. It's gotten later than they realized and they sense a change of mood. A gang of older men gathers around them.

"You kids got any money?" one man asks.

"We don't have anything," a young man replies.

"We're students from the university," another one explains. "We're down here studying the situation. I mean…"

One of the older men laughs, a stiff, mirthless laugh, more like a cough. It's a hot summer night but suddenly it feels cold.

"We're trying to figure out if there's anything we can do to help you," a third young man says. It's Tommy Douglas.

There's another laugh. Several of the men join in. Then the laughter fades out and there's an awkward silence. The students shift uneasily from foot to foot as the older men eye them suspiciously.

"Sonny, you can't do anything to help us, there's nothing you can do," one grizzled old man, dressed in the characteristic overalls and striped cap of a rail-roader, says finally. "But go back to that school of yours, and work, and see that this doesn't happen again."

∽

Flash back a year.

Brandon College had sent two candidates to Weyburn, a prosperous city of five thousand people, for the opening at Calvary Baptist Church: best friends Tommy Douglas and Stanley Knowles. The congregation of a hundred and forty liked them both, but ultimately the job went to Tommy. Knowles wound up in Winnipeg at the First Baptist Church, and became active in politics around the same time Tommy did, though it took him longer to get elected.

Tommy's annual salary was $1,800 which, supplemented by Irma's earnings from teaching piano, would have allowed them to live quite comfortably, except that Tommy kept giving money away – a pattern he'd follow the rest of his life.

Tommy and Irma rented a small apartment on Second Avenue and quickly threw themselves into the life of the church and the community. They skated and curled, attended concerts and lectures, joined clubs. At home, Tommy and Irma, on clarinet and piano, amused themselves with makeshift concerts when he wasn't writing sermons or doing papers for the correspondence courses he was taking from McMaster University.

He helped raise money for a civic swimming pool and, sitting down carelessly on a wooden bench at the edge of the pool in his swimsuit, earned the nickname Slivers.

The Reverend Douglas liked his little jokes. He had let the Calvary congregation know about his impending wedding by announcing, "Next Sunday we're going to have a new pianist." When an old girlfriend came to visit, he told Irma: "I think you'll like her. But it's a little difficult. She's very hard of hearing." Then he went down to the station to pick the young woman up, telling her, "Irma's a marvelous person, but there's just one thing. You'll have to raise your voice; she's quite deaf." Tommy made the introductions, then stepped back grinning and left the two women to shout at each other.

Sometimes the joke was on him, though. Already at work on his master's degree in sociology, Tommy spent many hours at the Weyburn mental hospital studying the patients. One afternoon he stayed later than usual and had a devil of a time convincing a new orderly that he wasn't a patient himself.

∞

"Here was the least common denominator of nature," W.O. Mitchell wrote in his wonderful novel *Who Has Seen the Wind*, "the skeleton requirements simply of land and sky – Saskatchewan prairie."

Saskatchewan, of course, is more than just land and sky, though both are so vast, and seemingly so essential, that they dominate, not just the landscape but the minds of people who live there.

In 1930, the province of Saskatchewan was only twenty-five years old. Of course, native Indians had lived on its prairies and parkland and in northern woods for thousands of years, but except for a handful of explorers and fur traders, it wasn't until Confederation in 1867 that outsiders began to take Saskatchewan seriously as a place to settle. And it wasn't until the arrival of the North-West Mounted Police and the railway, a few years later, that the floodgates to wide-scale immigration were opened. By the time Tommy Douglas arrived in Weyburn, the population had peaked at around 925,000, and Saskatchewan had become the third most populous province in the country. Many of the immigrants were from central and eastern Europe, creating an ethnic mix that was much like that of the North End Winnipeg where he'd grown up.

Wheat was king. Using irrigation and other modern agricultural methods, European farmers turned the semi-arid southern Saskatchewan prairie, known as the Palliser Triangle, into the best wheat-growing land in the world, and the province's economy rose and fell on grain prices on world markets.

The dependence on wheat became Saskatchewan's ruination in the thirties during the Great Depression. The price of wheat went into the toilet, freefalling from $1.60 a bushel to below 40 cents. Mother Nature rubbed salt into the wounds with a devastating drought and insect infestations – very little of this cheap wheat could be grown, and what was grown was attacked and destroyed by plagues of grasshoppers. Things went from bad to worse. Without water, farmers couldn't even raise chickens and grow gardens. As Tommy noted, "That meant that people did not have garden vegetables, chickens, cream, butter and eggs that a farmer would normally have. It was more than just a loss of income; it was a loss of sustenance." Fertile land was turned into a desert; precious topsoil turned to dust and whipped into the air at the whim of Saskatchewan's ever-present winds. Dust storms were so thick they turned the sky black, giving rise to the often-repeated expression, "The Dirty Thirties." Housewives put damp towels around windows and doors to keep out the dust.

This was the Saskatchewan Tommy and Irma Douglas came to in 1930, just as the reality of the Depression was starting to sink in.

∞

In addition to Calvary, Reverend Douglas's responsibilities included a church in the nearby town of Stoughton and services in surrounding rural areas, which made for very busy Sundays. There were also weddings, funerals, visits to the sick, and individual-counselling.

The new young preacher was an instant hit. Everyone liked him. Older members of the congregation began comparing him to Charles Haddon Spurgeon, the famous British "prince of preachers" whose sermons were published in best-selling books. Younger people liked him for his "down to earth" style.

"Whatever Tommy did drew a crowd," remembered one of his young parishioners, Babs Robertson. "Both he and Irma were so hospitable and filled with fun. What I remember most is how much fun it was. You never felt in awe of Tommy. You felt that he was one of you. You never felt that because he was a minister he was above you. He was down to earth."

Many of Tommy's activities as a minister were directed toward teenagers. In addition to the normal Sunday school, he involved children of church members in dramatics, athletics, and social clubs. Sometimes he was called on for service above and beyond the call of duty.

One Monday morning, with Tommy still basking in the good feelings of his Sunday sermons, he had a phone call from the police magistrate.

"I have eleven boys coming up before me this morning for juvenile delinquency," the judge explained. "They're constant repeaters. I hate to send them to the Industrial School in Regina – it's pretty grim there – but I don't know what to do with them, and I haven't much choice unless somebody will do something about it. I was wondering if you'd come down to watch the proceedings."

Tommy went to court and was disturbed by what he saw and heard. The boys all lived in a shanty community on the outskirts of town, and many were from broken families who had given up on them. They'd been into all sorts of trouble, from truancy and fighting, to shoplifting, pickpocketing, and outright theft. They were scruffy, in dirty, torn clothing, their hair long, greasy and tangled. Before he knew what he was doing, Tommy had spoken up and had the judge commit them to his care.

"I took them home," he remembered. "To march in with eleven ragamuffins was quite a sight, and my wife, to whom I'd been married for less than a year, just about went home to her mother. She was a good sport, though."

Together, they got the kids fed, and then Tommy was on the phone to some of his parishioners with children of their own to round up clothes. The boys had baths and haircuts, and the older ones were lined up with odd jobs for pocket money. And the young minister, helped out by some of the boys in his congregation, did everything he could to keep the tough kids busy and out of trouble.

"One of the first significant things we noticed was that these boys didn't know how to play," he said. "They could fight at the drop of a hat and knew everything except the Marquis of Queensbury rules. They could pick a lock. They could get into a building and out again, and you'd never know how they got there. But they couldn't play games."

Tommy's gang of boys were regular angels during the week while he was able to keep a watchful eye on them, but they tended to backslide on Sundays, when he'd be busy all day. He came home from one of his rural postings one Sunday and found a very irate store-keeper waiting for him: the boys had broken into his shop and made off with cigarettes and boxes of choco-lates. Tommy had a good idea of where the boys might be and tracked them down to a smoke-filled shack where they were gorging on chocolate. Because he had evening service to prepare for, he didn't have time for more than laying down the law and ordering them to report to his study afterwards.

For years afterwards, Tommy loved telling this story: "So they were all at church that Sunday evening, and sat through the service, looking as innocent as angels; then after the service they trooped into the study and I gave them my very best lecture. How they had let me down, had let down the other young people in the church who had worked with them and tried to help them." There was nothing left to do but turn them back to the judge, he said ruefully.

"They began to sniff and cry, and the tears flowed."

They promised they wouldn't stray again, and Tommy agreed to give them another chance. On their way out, one boy, Reggie, stopped. Tommy remem-bered that "he was the toughest of the lot, he could pick a lock with a hairpin, he had all the aptitudes for a

criminal, and was very courageous. He would fight anything, any size. He was thin and wiry; he looked like a
terrier. He stopped and he said, 'Mr. Douglas, I'm terribly sorry for what we've done. I'm so sorry. I want to
give you back your things.'

"And he handed me back my watch, my penknife,
my fountain pen, and a half a dozen other things he'd
stolen off my desk while I was giving my ten-cent lecture."

Increasingly, as the effects of the Depression took
hold, there would be fewer lighthearted moments like
this one and more heartbreaking ones.

The churches of Weyburn had sent out a plea for
help to churches in parts of the country where the
Depression was yet to be felt as strongly, and help was
coming. From British Columbia rolled railway cars full
of fruit and vegetables. There were no buyers for the
produce and, rather than see it rot, growers donated it
to feed the hungry. From Ontario came boxcars of
clothing, both used and new, donated by storekeepers
cleaning out old stock. People lined up, and Tommy
and the town's other ministers rolled up their sleeves
and scooped fruits and vegetables into sacks. They also
distributed clothing to anyone who asked for it.

But some people were too proud to ask.

"How're you fixed for bedding?" Tommy asked a
woman one morning as she was leaving church. She
and her husband had once been prosperous farmers,
and Tommy knew they'd be unlikely to seek help for
themselves or their half dozen children. But the sharp-
eyed minister noticed how threadbare their clothes had
become.

Her eyes filled up with tears. "Mr. Douglas, I haven't got a decent sheet in the place. We're patched and patched and I just don't know how I'm going to get by."

"How are the youngsters for clothing?" Tommy inquired.

The woman could barely talk. "Well, they haven't got any winter underwear, so I've been trying to make some out of flour sacks."

"Just stay behind and we'll fix it up," Tommy said, putting his hand on her arm and giving her a reassuring smile.

Tommy grew increasingly impatient with the limitations of the church. "The religion of tomorrow will be less concerned with dogmas of theology and more concerned with the social welfare of humanity," he wrote in a magazine article. "When one sees the church spending its energies on the assertion of antiquated dogmas but dumb as an oyster to the poverty and misery all around, we can't help but recognize the need for a new interpretation of Christianity."

That kind of thinking was heresy to many clergymen. At a church convention, when Tommy proposed a resolution echoing those sentiments, an older minister insisted the division in classes was part of God's plan, so the rich could learn charity and the poor could learn gratitude. The church, this man argued, shouldn't worry about people's condition in this world but rather should prepare them for the next one.

∞

Bad as things were in Weyburn, Tommy was shaken even harder by his experiences in Chicago, where he spent the summer of 1931 doing graduate work. He was part of a group of University of Chicago students sent to study conditions in the city's massive hobo jungle along the railroad tracks. It was a virtual city in itself, with an estimated seventy thousand occupants living in boxcars, lean-tos and junked vehicles, many of them reduced to begging and stealing to keep alive.

"These were not just bums and hobos," he recalled. "They were decent boys who had come from the same kind of home I had. The only difference was that I had a job and they didn't. That shook me."

Among the hobos were people from all sorts of backgrounds, including skilled workers, bank clerks, university students, people with law and medical degrees. So much for God's plan for the classes! And what was just as shocking as the desperate plight these men found themselves in was the stark fact that the economic system had let them down. This wasn't a quirk of nature, as the Saskatchewan drought was, but a man-made disaster. "I'd studied socialism and syndicalism and communism and capitalism," Tommy would later tell an interviewer, "but I'd never sat down and honestly asked myself what was wrong with the economic system."

In Chicago, he also found time to meet with Norman Thomas, the leader of the U.S. Socialist Party, and to attend some party meetings, which further disillusioned him. "At the first one," he remembered, "they sat around debating whether after the revolution people would eat in their own homes or come to dining kitchens for communal meals." It disgusted Tommy that "the fact that people didn't have anything to eat didn't seem to bother them at all."

Before he knew it, he was on his feet shooting off his mouth: 'What are you going to do *now*?'"

The experience soured him on political purists and theorists who felt they should stand back and let things get so bad revolution would be sparked through spontaneous combustion. "You don't press a button and an old society disappears and a new one is born next morning at seven o'clock," he argued. "Society is changed organically; you slough off the old and the new takes its place. You do what you can for people and work for change."

Tommy shook his head with exasperation. "I've no patience with people who want to sit back and talk about a blueprint for society and do nothing about it. I got that in Chicago."

∞

Back home in Weyburn, Tommy got busy organizing the unemployed, setting up an odd-job agency that put idle men to work doing household repairs. He went to city hall to press for increases in relief rates. Businessmen were alarmed, and some began calling Tommy a "Red," a dangerous radical. By his own admission, he was a nuisance.

Some people just refused to accept what was plain as the noses on their faces, clinging to the belief that anyone who wanted to work could find a job, that only layabouts needed relief.

A member of the Calvary congregation chided him about his organizing work. A well-dressed lawyer, he was treasurer of the Young Fellows, a prominent businessman's group. "I just can't understand it," he told Tommy. "Why do you get mixed up with that crowd?"

"What do you know about them?" Tommy shot back.

"Well, I see them when I go down the street...."

"Do you know anything about them, really?"

"I suppose not."

"You see people in your office who've got some money or they wouldn't be coming here. They're concerned about money matters, setting up their estate or buying or selling property. Have you ever actually seen the conditions in the poorer part of this city?"

"I've lived in this city for twenty-five years," the lawyer protested. "I lived here before you came here."

"Yes, but you don't see it as it is now."

The upshot of this conversation was that Tommy took his friend on a guided tour of Weyburn's underside. They went to homes where there was no coal for heat, where the kids had no shoes and hadn't had milk for a week. They saw people sick but with no money for a doctor, a pregnant woman beside herself because she had no layette or diapers for her baby. And they saw boys who'd been playing sports for the high school team a year earlier now idle because they couldn't afford university and had no jobs.

When they got back to his office, the lawyer was close to tears. "I wouldn't have believed it," he said, shaking his head. "I know this might happen in the east side of London but for it to be happening in the town where I live. I'm ashamed that I don't know this."

Tommy went home feeling good about himself that night, but by morning the feeling had dissipated. For every person whose eyes he might open, there were hundreds of others who refused to see. He remembered the haunted, hungry plea of the man in Chicago's hobo jungle, "see that this doesn't happen again."

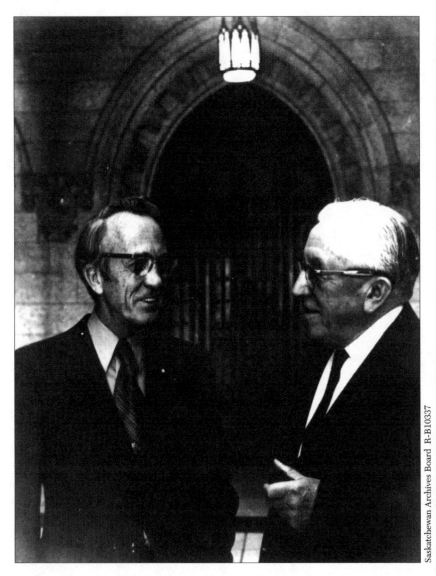

Saskatchewan radicals Douglas and Coldwell stand together in Ottawa in 1971, almost forty years after they changed the course of Canadian history.

5

Trading the Pulpit for Politics

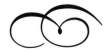

One Saturday morning in 1932, Major Coldwell receives a letter – there was Saturday mail delivery in those days! – from J. S. Woodsworth, Tommy Douglas's former pastor, who is now a Labour member of Parliament.

Coldwell, a teacher and high school principal in Regina and a member of city council, is a leader in provincial left-wing movements and a popular radio personality. He usually uses his initials, M.J., because his given name, Major, makes it sound like he's a military man, and Coldwell, a pacifist with a smooth British accent and an engaging manner, is anything but. Tommy Douglas had written to Woodsworth for advice, expressing his frustration with the lack of action on social issues, and the older man thought he and Coldwell, who had also written to him with similar thoughts, should get together. He wrote to both men suggesting just that.

Coldwell reads Woodsworth's letter twice, first quickly, then more slowly. Then, since there's no school today, Coldwell asks his fifteen-year-old son Jack if he'd like to go for a drive in the country, and the two set out to Weyburn. Directed to the Baptist Church "manse," a bungalow the Douglases moved to the previous fall, Coldwell knocks on the door, which is answered by a young woman.

"Is your father at home?" Coldwell inquires.

Irma Douglas blushes. "No, but you'll find my husband at the church."

Tommy's working on his sermon for the next day. He puts it aside and, like two teenaged boys swapping hockey cards, he and Coldwell plunge into a political discussion.

They hit it off immediately, becoming fast friends. They have plenty to talk about.

Depression and drought had been battering Weyburn, and all of Saskatchewan, since Tommy arrived to take up his church duties at Calvary Baptist Church two years earlier.

The Conservative governments in Regina and Ottawa seemed powerless to combat either the huge economic problems besetting the province and country, which had left over a million people out of work, or

Mother Nature's practical joke, which was turning the Prairies into a dustbowl. Prime Minister R.B. Bennett "was doing all the wrong things about the Depression, just as (U.S. President) Hoover had done," Tommy observed.

Things were particularly bad on the Prairies. Saskatchewan had plummeted from fourth wealthiest province to the poorest. In the Weyburn area, 95 per cent of farmers were on relief, which meant they had little to spend in town. Businesses closed and workers lost their jobs. The beds of Weyburn's hospital were empty as the town's impoverished sick stayed home.

As a minister of the cloth, Tommy Douglas felt powerless as he saw his parishioners suffer. Prayer wasn't enough, he was certain. Action was required – but what?

He had taken small actions on the home front, such as organizing the unemployed into the Weyburn Labour Association, only to meet hostility on the part of the city's establishment. It didn't seem enough. Political action, on the provincial if not the federal level, seemed to be the inevitable answer – but, again, exactly what?

Then came the troubles at Estevan.

The coal-mining town some eighty kilometres southeast of Weyburn was rocked by a strike in September 1931, shortly after Tommy's return from Chicago. Miners, already poorly paid, dug their heels in when mine owners cut their pay further, knowing there were plenty of unemployed men willing to take their jobs. Their situation was aggravated by the loss of part-time jobs on farms, with which they normally supplemented their incomes. The Mine Workers Union called a strike September 8, and a hostile government and press railed against the workers. The spectre of the Bolshevik Revolution was summoned up, just as it had been in the Winnipeg General Strike a dozen years earlier. A horrified public focused on the presence of communists in the union, on "outside agitators," obscuring the issues of low wages and cruel working conditions. Only the United Farmers of Canada, a Saskatchewan group with radical leadership, was sympathetic.

When Tommy and Irma paid a visit to Estevan and the nearby village of Bienfait, they were shocked by the company-owned shacks the miners and their families lived in, and the company store system that kept them constantly in debt. Tommy preached against these conditions the following Sunday and organized a food collection for the strikers and their families. The mine owners complained to the Calvary deacons, and Tommy's reputation as a Red and a troublemaker grew.

Things went from bad to worse on September 29, when the miners attempted to stage a parade on Estevan's main street. Mounties reinforced by private police hired by the mine owners – another echo of the Winnipeg strike – grew nervous and attacked the marchers. Twenty-three people, some of them merely bystanders, were injured; three of them died.

Tommy grew increasingly frustrated. He thought about his work with the unemployed, and thought also of the support local farmers and farm organizations had given the striking mine workers. He started to wonder about the possibility of bringing farm and labour together to work for mutual concerns. What was there to lose? These were the thoughts on his mind when he wrote to Woodsworth.

∞

The meeting of M.J. and Tommy was a marriage made in heaven. A quiet-spoken, gentlemanly man, Coldwell was, as Tommy himself described his new mentor, "a flaming radical" compared to the young clergyman. "He was the most dynamic fellow I ever met. You see, people were losing their homes, being put off their farms, going *hungry*. M.J. was outraged by these conditions. He and George Williams (a farm leader) roused the Prairies, became the centre of protest against these *unnecessary* hardships of the people."

Over the next couple of years, a tremendous amount of political activity would occur, culminating in the creation of the Co-Operative Commonwealth Federation (CCF), a national left-wing party. Tommy wouldn't always be directly involved. He still had his congregation to look after, his graduate studies, and his young family – daughter Shirley was born in April 1934 – but every step the movement took would eventually have an impact on his future.

Tommy had been becoming more and more frustrated with the confines of the church, and had been gravitating toward a path of political action. But it was his meeting with Coldwell, more than anything else, that set him irrevocably in motion along that path.

The immediate result of that meeting was the organization of a labour party in Weyburn, with

Tommy as president, soon linked to a provincewide group headed by Coldwell. But on July 27, 1932, the farmers movement, in the form of George Williams's United Farmers, and the labour movement, in the form of M.J. Coldwell's Independent Labour Party, came together to create the Farmer-Labour Party, the Saskatchewan link in what would a year later blossom into the national party called the CCF. This historic marriage occurred in an empty building on the Regina Exhibition Grounds, while outside the annual Saskatchewan Exhibition swirled around them, and children shouted in excitement from the midway. Coldwell was chosen party leader; George Williams, the dour, abrasive leader of the United Farmers of Canada, was made chairman of the party's council.

Tommy missed the big moment. He was off in Winnipeg taking an economics course required for his master's studies. In his absence, he was elected a representative to the new party's council. But being a political candidate was still the farthest thing from his mind. Tommy missed another important meeting the following month too: the final preparatory conference, in Calgary, leading up the formation of the CCF. The name the conference chose was based on a tried and true phrase in left-wing ideology, "co-operative commonwealth," but, when he heard it, Tommy thought it was "an awful mouthful."

The next summer, when the CCF held its founding convention in Regina, selecting Woodsworth as national leader, Tommy missed most of that, too, only managing to get there for the last of the three days of meetings, but he told friends it was "the finest thing I have ever seen." He was particularly enthusiastic about the soon-to-become-famous Regina Manifesto issued at the convention, which called for public health insurance, unemployment insurance and pension plans, expansion of Crown corporations, including into transportation, communication, and banks, and adoption of a Canadian constitution with an entrenched charter of rights. These are all well-established parts of Canadian life now but were radical ideas in the thirties.

The manifesto also vowed to eradicate capitalism, probably its most famous pledge and the one that made the CCF vulnerable to criticism as a thinly veiled form of communism.

The manifesto had been drafted by a group of young Ontario intellectuals who'd gathered around Woodsworth, but their words rang true to the farm-based Saskatchewan socialists who had seen the capitalist system fail them in dramatic fashion. "To me, it was a good pragmatic document," Tommy would reflect later. "I've often wondered what all the fuss was about."

Tommy's own view of socialism gradually took shape during this period. As is often the case when people come to new ideas, he was torn by conflicting sentiments. On one hand, as a man deeply influenced by the Bible and Christian thinking, he strongly believed in the value of the individual, and this made grassroots populism attractive to him. Political decisions, he felt, should be made by the people affected, not politicians, bureaucrats, and backroom fixers. On the other hand, his intellectual training drove him to abhor the irrational and to embrace rational solutions.

The Depression was proof aplenty that the economic system of capitalism, with its emphasis on the "wisdom of the marketplace," had gone off its hinges, and "free enterprise" was just a dirty joke. "It's every man for himself, as the elephant said when he danced among the chickens," was how Tommy wryly put it.

The solution, it seemed to this young minister, was a form of social engineering, where social and economic problems would be studied scientifically and rational decisions made by experts.

This reliance on planning and expertise, which can so easily degenerate into what George Orwell, in his novel *1984*, called "Big Brother," also led Tommy to a brief flirtation with the dubious science of eugenics – controlled human breeding.

For his master's degree work in sociology from McMaster, he was studying "the subnormal family" and had identified a group of "immoral or nonmoral women" in the Weyburn area – the dozen women had produced ninety-five children and over a hundred grandchildren. Studying this brood, he found many examples of venereal and other diseases, poor performance in school, illegitimacy, crime, and other examples of "moral delinquency."

In the thesis, he wrote "the subnormal family presents the most appalling of all family problems.... Surely, the continued policy of allowing the subnormal family to bring into the world large numbers of individuals to fill our jails and our mental institutions, and to live upon charity, is one of consummate folly." He proposed sterilization for "mentally defective" and incurably diseased people. Not a very Christian view, nor one that would win much favour with leftists, or rational people in general, in this day and age. But in 1933, such thinking had become popular.

Eugenics lost its appeal for many people after it was embraced by Germany's Nazis, who, as part of their larger plan to build a master race, used enforced sterilization against a wide variety of people they found undesirable. Not surprisingly, by the time Tommy was premier and minister of health of Saskatchewan, and in a position to put some of his earlier ideas into practice, he'd changed his mind.

∞

Although Tommy had no real desire to run for office, when a provincial election was called for June 1934, he was pressured by his Farmer-Labour colleagues into the campaign. The Conservatives, whose efforts at dealing with the effects of Depression and drought had been inept, were clearly doomed, and the Liberals, under the popular James Gardiner, were likely to form the next government. In Weyburn, the Grits had what seemed to be an unbeatable candidate in the form of Hugh Eaglesham, a much-loved family doctor "who had brought half the people in our community into the world," as Tommy put it. "And so nobody wanted to run." But duty called and Tommy answered.

Totally inexperienced in practical politics, Tommy, by his own admission, wasn't very effective. He conducted the campaign "like a university professor giving a course in sociology. I had charts and so on, and I'm sure half the people didn't know what I was talking about."

Compared to the campaigns of today, Tommy's 1934 venture was strictly a shoestring operation – and broken shoestrings at that. There were no campaign contributions, certainly not from corporate donors, just the loose change that would be collected by passing a hat at rallies and meetings. The campaign car was an old Model A Ford Tommy and Irma had found in the garage when they bought their house and had managed to make roadworthy. "You'd be very fortunate if you got enough to pay your gas bill for the next meeting," Tommy remembered. Just the same, he managed to get to 120 meetings, visiting many of the communities in his riding several times.

The new party also ran into stiff opposition to some of its policies, like some of the pledges in the Regina Manifesto. Because of a plank that called for partial socialization of farmland, many farmers thought they'd lose their land if Farmer-Labour won. Hostility to socialism by the Roman Catholic Church was another obstacle. Despite all this, Tommy and his supporters were incurable optimists and convinced themselves they would win. After all, some two thousand people turned out to hear Tommy and Woodsworth at a Weyburn rally. They were also buoyed by the CCF's showing in the British Columbia election late in 1933, just a few months after the party's formal launch, in which six members were elected and, more importantly, the fledgling party won a third of the popular vote.

Tommy's third-place loss, therefore, and the party's capture of only five seats in the legislature, were big disappointments.

Just the same, the campaign didn't exactly light a fire under Tommy Douglas the politician. Having done his duty, he wanted only to get on with his life. He had offers from other churches, including one in Milwaukee, but the academic life also appealed to him and, having finally gotten his M.A., he was thinking seriously of moving his family to Chicago so he could pursue his Ph.D. full time. Before he had a chance to make up his mind, though, an immovable object and an irresistible force collided to change his life forever.

A federal election was looming for 1935, but Tommy had no interest in running. "You can 'include me out,'" he said. "I've done my job, and there must be somebody else around here who can run." He put the idea out of his mind and went off to Chicago for a summer of study.

That's the way things would have stayed except for what must have been divine intervention in the form of a butt-inski superintendent from the Baptist Church. His disapproval of Tommy's having run in the provincial election was apparent, but when he canvassed Calvary parishioners, he found few who objected to the young minister's political activities. He had come to scold Tommy, but decided not to. But he couldn't resist getting in a dig.

"Your people don't mind it, and if they don't mind it, of course I'm not going to say anything about it," the church official told Tommy. "Except this is to be the last. You're not to run again."

As it happened, Calvary was a self-supporting church and didn't need the Baptist organization's blessing for anything it did, but Tommy knew the superintendent could blackball him at other churches. And, as it happened, he was considering an offer from Strathcona Baptist Church in Edmonton, which had called just the previous day. To his surprise, his visitor encouraged him to take the job.

"I suggest you go there and carry on with your university work at the same time," he said. "I think that's the best thing for you to do."

"Many people here have been pressing me to run again," Tommy said. "I don't want to run. On the other hand, I've seen the party build up and I hate to walk out and leave it."

"Leave it," the superintendent warned. "If you don't leave it, and if you don't stay out of politics, you'll never get another church in Canada, and I'll see to it. The board has given me authority."

Those were fighting words to Tommy Douglas. "You've just given the CCF a candidate," he replied.

And his future was sealed.

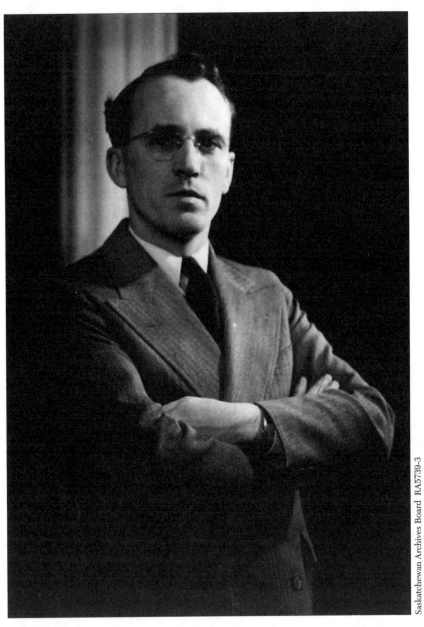

Tommy Douglas is elected to Parliament in 1935 and quickly establishes himself as a sharp-tongued debater and a critic of the government. "So this is Parliament? Pardon me, I thought it was a kindergarten."

6

Member of Parliament

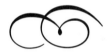

Weyburn, a cold night in late September, 1935, just a few weeks before the federal election. A huge crowd, almost seven thousand people, has turned out at the arena, a big drafty hockey rink, to hear the MP for area, Liberal Ed Young, take on the CCF newcomer, the Reverend T.C. Douglas.

Young's thin, squeaky voice is no match for Tommy's trained one, used to barn-dance oratory. Nor can the MP match his young opponent for brass. In response to Young's attacks on the CCF, Tommy sneers that the Liberal stands merely for "survival of the slickest."

But the sucker punch comes moments after Young flaunts a copy of Tommy's new campaign brochure, waving it in the air and exclaiming, "I don't know what all the fuss is about. There's nothing in this pamphlet, and it needn't bother anyone." He reads parts of it to the audience in a sarcastic tone.

Tommy happens to know the pamphlet in Young's hand has been stolen – and so do most of the people in the audience, fidgeting restlessly in their heavy coats. The pamphlets haven't been released yet, and two nights earlier there was a break-in at the print shop. Just yesterday, Tommy and an RCMP constable went to visit Young's campaign manager, J.J. McCruden, at the school in the village of McTaggart, where Young is principal. With giggling school kids gawking nearby, McCruden bowed his head in shame and admitted the theft.

"Any man who would stoop to such methods is unfit to be a teacher of the youth of this country," Tommy tells the hushed arena. "And any man who would make use of stolen property on a political platform is unfit to represent the people of this constituency in Parliament!"

The crowd explodes, the rafters of the arena ringing with cheers and boos. Young is shaking his fist at Tommy, and Principal McCruden leaps onto the platform, fire in his eye. A bulky man standing six feet, two inches (1.8 metres), he looms over Tommy and threatens to knock his head off. Several husky farmers jump over the railing and gather around the platform, one of them pointing menacingly at the principal and shouting, "Don't you dare touch him."

Says Tommy: "It was a great wind-up."

∞

Tommy Douglas's victory in the 1935 federal election, which launched a forty-four-year-long career as an elected politician, almost didn't happen. He won by a mere 301 votes, and only after a dirty campaign that relied on the tricks of an early-day "spin doctor" and almost got Tommy expelled from the CCF.

Even before his decision to run, Tommy had become a national leader of the party. At the CCF convention in Winnipeg the previous summer, Woodsworth had asked Tommy, then not quite thirty, to head up the party's youth wing in order to quell a revolt from the left. Tommy became convinced that the agitators were communists intent on taking over the CCF or breaking it up.

The national profile that presidency of the CCF youth wing gave him, along with his local reputation as a troublemaker, made Tommy the ideal candidate to go up against Ed Young. The veteran Liberal MP had developed a reputation as an errand boy for big business and gave Tommy a great opportunity to score points when C.L. Burton, millionaire president of Simpson's department stores, paid a mid-campaign visit, parking his private railway car at the Weyburn station for all to see. Burton had just made headlines in Regina where he proposed that jobless men be put in army training camps.

Young had also lodged his foot squarely in his mouth with a careless comment in Parliament that "Canadians must learn to accept a lower standard of living." It was a reasonable thing to say, perhaps, at the height of the Great Depression, but certainly not what the voters wanted to hear, and Tommy made Young eat those words.

After his campaign started making use of the Young quote, Tommy asked a farmer one day if he'd decided who to vote for. "I know who I'm *not* going to vote for," the farmer replied, "that fellow who says we have to settle down to a lower standard of living." Tommy was impressed. There was obviously political value in simplicity.

It was Dan Grant who seized on the Young quote and persuaded Tommy to make hay with it. A political gadfly who had cut his teeth working for the Ku Klux Klan during its brief rise to popularity in Saskatchewan in the twenties, Grant had wound up with a government job in Weyburn but was fired when Gardiner and his Grits came to power. With time on his hands and all sorts of ideas, plus a desire for revenge against the Liberals, he signed on with the Douglas campaign as a driver and general go-fer. A spiritualist and tea-leaf reader, the dapper Grant in his bowler hat and high collar was an oddball by any standards, but he had the instincts of a shark when it came to campaigning. In addition to talking Tommy into making use of Young's "lower standard of living" comment, Grant was the one who insisted a charge be laid after the theft of the pamphlets.

And when principal McCruden confessed the theft, it was Grant who "made a great fuss about it," Tommy remembered. "To me it didn't matter at all, but to Grant, this was terrific."

Dan Grant also came up with the idea for "the silver bullet" raffle. When Tommy's old Model A Ford gave up the ghost, Grant sweet-talked a local car dealer into providing a brand new silver Hudson Terraplane on credit for use as a campaign car. On every stop, while Tommy worked the crowd, Grant sold tickets on the car at a buck a piece, raking in enough to pay off the car, which was raffled off at campaign's end, and to cover most travel expenses.

Gone were the professorial lectures Tommy had used in the 1934 campaign. Along with simplicity and the attention-grabbing gimmicks he learned from Dan Grant, Tommy added drama and humour, fashioning a political style out of his own experience: one part preacher, one part actor and orator, one part standup comic, one part Robert Burns. In short, he relaxed and learned to be himself on the stump.

"I began telling jokes," he recalled, "because those people needed entertainment. They looked so tired and frustrated and weary. The women particularly. They had all the back-breaking work to do. So I used to tell the jokes to cheer them up.

"And when they're laughing, they're listening."

Tommy needed a sense of humour. As campaign passions intensified, he had to have a lock put on the gas cap of his shiny new car after several attempts at sabotage with sugar and sand, and one evening, when he and Grant had a flat tire, they were dismayed to discover all the nuts on the back wheels of the Silver Bullet had been loosened.

Things really got ugly at a meeting at a school in the village of Odessa when a gang of young men who'd been sitting quietly in the packed auditorium suddenly started shouting and heckling, then charged the stage.

Tommy noted quickly that there was no back door, then saw Calvary deacon Ted Stinson, his campaign manager, take off his jacket and start to roll up his sleeves. The former lightweight champ of Manitoba picked up a water jug, smashed it against a table to give himself a weapon, and shouted out: "If you come up here, you're going to get hurt."

Just then, another group of young men, CCF supporters, arrived at the door and things calmed down. "Having any trouble, Tommy?" one of them asked.

"Not now."

The stillborn violence of the moment shook Tommy, reminding him of that never-to-be-forgotten afternoon of the Winnipeg Strike riot, of the trouble in Estevan and, even more recently, the riot in Regina on July 1 that year, when police had attacked a peaceful rally organized by unemployed men trekking to Ottawa to demand government changes. Tommy wasn't present, but he was in Regina the next day for a radio broadcast and heard vivid accounts from Dr. Hugh MacLean, a CCF activist who'd spent hours patching up victims of the police rampage, and it had strengthened his resolve.

But vandals, hooligans, and the police were nothing compared to the problems caused Tommy by Social Credit.

That political movement was championed by another preacher-turned-politician, "Bible Bill" Aberhart, a fundamentalist whose religious radio broadcasts had a big audience in Alberta. Aberhart and his Socreds, as they were dubbed, swept to power in Alberta in August 1935, less than two months before the federal election.

Fundamentally a conservative movement, Social Credit nevertheless sounded a lot like the CCF on the surface, and, in politically charged 1935, it was easy for voters to be confused about the differences between the two new parties. Both, after all, attacked the two old-line parties and banks, Bay Street businessmen, and the "big interests" back East. The Saskatchewan situation became increasingly cloudy late that summer with the news that the victorious Aberhart was looking eastward.

The CCF brain trust took a cautious approach. Party leaders M.J. Coldwell and George Williams issued a joint statement emphasizing that Social Credit was a capitalist party but pledging that CCF members of Parliament would try to thwart any federal efforts to stifle Aberhart's economic experiments.

But in Weyburn, Tommy Douglas and his supporters worried that a Social Credit candidate could split the protest vote, giving the Liberals' Ed Young a free ride.

What followed was a piece of political sleight of hand worthy of Watergate, not illegal but far from proper. It got Tommy into a world of trouble – but also may have been the final trick that got him elected.

The way Tommy, campaign manager Ted Stinson, and Dan Grant saw it, even if a real Social Credit candidate didn't emerge, the Liberals might put up a phony one. Either way, the CCF would lose votes.

In early September, Stinson met with an Aberhart lieutenant in Moose Jaw and won an agreement that the new Alberta premier would endorse Tommy if he could win local Social Credit support.

Tommy's first move was to issue a statement, echoing the one from Coldwell and Williams but going a bit further: if he was elected, he told *The Weyburn Review*, he was "prepared to initiate and support legislation...which would make possible the Social Credit system being operated in any province caring to do so."

Then, Stinson, Grant, and some others set up a bogus Weyburn Social Credit Association. The Liberals did the same thing, offering a CCF supporter named Eric Mackay $2,000 to be its candidate. He turned them down, but they found another political wannabe, Morton Fletcher, to pose as a Socred and get in the race.

On September 28, Tommy addressed the Social Credit group his people had formed and was able to read aloud a telegram from Aberhart pledging his support. The CCF had beaten the Liberals at the Socred shell game.

But that wasn't the end of the story.

CCF officials, from Woodsworth on down, were becomingly increasingly uneasy about collaborating with an enemy party. And in Regina, Williams and his supporters hit the roof when they got wind of posters supporting Tommy and bearing the name of the "Weyburn CCF-Social Credit Committee." Things got even tenser when a Socred official from Alberta appeared on a platform with Tommy, and *The Regina Leader Post* reported Tommy had "officially declared his willingness to support the Social Credit platform 100 per cent," a distortion of his earlier statement.

Tommy was called on the carpet October 9, just five days before the election. He was summoned to Regina to meet with five top members of the CCF, led by Williams, in a meeting room at the Hotel Saskatchewan. His accusers had a copy of the offending poster and, even worse, the telegram confirming Tommy "as a Social Credit candidate."

"You have very successfully crucified the provincial organization," Williams growled.

"You're wrong if you think I'm supporting a capitalist movement," Tommy shot back. "I merely promised to give Social Credit a free hand and support legislation to do so. That's exactly what George and M.J. said we should do." He glared at the frowning Williams, who snatched up the offending poster and shook it in his fist.

"Who issued this?"

"Our joint committee."

"How did you arrange for the speaker?"

"We wrote and asked for a man to repudiate this man Fletcher."

"And you had this man sent from Alberta?"

"Yes."

At this point, Dr. MacLean, an ally of Coldwell's and an elder statesman of the party, interrupted: "Communists have endorsed me. I am not a communist."

"Did you do this because you felt you couldn't win without Social Credit?" asked another of the interrogators.

"Social Credit doesn't amount to a row of pins," Tommy scoffed.

"Then why not go on a straight CCF program?"

"We are," Tommy insisted. "I am the CCF candidate...and the Social Credit forces have the right to endorse me and a joint committee has the right to issue literature.... All I did was promise to give Aberhart a hand."

Then the cocky young preacher did something the Manitoba lightweight boxing champion probably would have avoided: he led with his chin. "Whatever action the executive takes does not affect me."

He was wrong, and escaped immediate expulsion from the party only on the insistence of MacLean. Williams and the others wanted him out, but the doctor persuaded them to hear first from Coldwell, who hadn't been able to make it to the meeting. The next day, Coldwell threatened to resign if Tommy was disciplined. Ejecting the Weyburn candidate "would have regrettable repercussions for the whole movement," he argued. But Coldwell did order there be no further consorting with the enemy without an OK from the party's top brass, and Tommy himself squeaked out of his tight corner with a light knuckle rapping.

Four days later, Tommy won his narrow victory. Morton Fletcher, the Liberal-supported "Socred," could only muster 362 votes. But it seemed clear that, without Tommy's claim to Social Credit support, Fletcher would have done better – at Tommy's expense.

Years later, he rationalized the deception this way: "Here was a mob of people, farmers, small businessmen, railway workers, who knew that something was wrong...and wanted to support something. And they didn't give a tinker's damn about all of the fine points."

Tommy, Irma, and baby Shirley spent the Christmas holidays in Winnipeg before setting off for

Ottawa. "Now, remember laddie," the elder Douglas told his son, "the working people have put a lot of trust in you, you must never let them down." Tommy had to return a month later for his father's funeral – he had died suddenly from a burst appendix, at fifty-seven. Then it was on to Ottawa again, and the beginning of what would be a much longer career in politics than he or anyone else expected.

Tommy Douglas would always be remembered as the preacher from Weyburn. He had resigned his position at Calvary Baptist Church, and, though he kept his status with the Baptists active and he occasionally delivered a guest sermon, he never worked as a minister again.

∞

Tommy fell quickly into the life of an MP. As a member of a marginal party, he could do little more than play the role of conscience to Parliament and prick in the side of the government, a role he relished. An MP's job is not all that different from a preacher's, after all – study and writing, meeting people and helping them with their problems, delivery of sermonlike speeches – and Tommy took to it readily.

The Liberals under Prime Minister William Lyon Mackenzie King had campaigned under the slogan "King or Chaos" and won a large majority. Although Woodsworth's party had fielded over a hundred candidates, it managed to send only eight members to Parliament, including party leader Woodsworth, Tommy, and M.J. – the only other Saskatchewan candidate to be elected – and Angus MacInnis from Vancouver. Angus's wife, Grace, who happened to be Woodsworth's daughter and would later be elected to Parliament herself, worked as caucus secretary, and the happy little crew was soon joined by David Lewis, a young lawyer from Montreal who had just returned from a term as Rhodes Scholar at Oxford and who became chief organizer for the party.

The Douglases were able to live comfortably on Tommy's $4,000-a-year salary, with an expense allowance of $2,000, and the free rail pass that came with the job meant frequent trips home. While Parliament was in session, they lived in a small Ottawa apartment, heading to Weyburn in the summer. As soon as Shirley was old enough to start school, though, Irma moved back to Weyburn with her to stay. At any rate, Tommy probably spent more time in the company of Coldwell than he did with his wife; the two men shared an office on the sixth floor of Parliament's Centre Block, and soon became the best and closest of friends, even rooming together after Irma's departure.

With a special interest in agriculture and, increasingly, foreign policy, Tommy quickly established himself as a sharp-tongued debater and a critic of the government. Denouncing the appointment of the head of a private grain handling company as chairman of the Canadian Wheat Board, he quipped it was like "putting a weasel in charge of the hen coop." Once, Jimmy Gardiner, who had left the Saskatchewan premiership to become Mackenzie King's agriculture minister, ridiculed his efforts for farmers, saying Tommy himself was no farmer. He shot back: "No. And I never laid an egg either, but I know more about omelets than most hens."

He scorned King's invitation to cross the floor, and, in an article he wrote for a magazine, he took his Liberal colleagues to task for ignoring the price of wheat but joining noisily in a debate on riding boundaries. "Feeding, clothing and caring for our people is of relatively little importance. Saving one's seat is of paramount importance. So this is Parliament? Pardon me, I thought it was a kindergarten."

In his maiden speech, Tommy lambasted the government for inaction on Italy's recent invasion of Ethiopia. He also rattled off a litany of concerns that would become recurrent themes during his years in Parliament and later: welfare, employment, unemployment insurance, farm produce prices, farm debt, health insurance.

"I had come fresh from the prairies where there was drought, poverty, and unemployment, and the Regina Riot left an indelible impression on me," he explained. "It was natural that I should want to speak about these things. It was also only natural...that I should feel a bit impatient with a government that seemed to be doing practically nothing about these problems."

The CCF MPs were often the subject of red-baiting, and Tommy particularly let himself open to that when he became vice-chairman of the League Against War and Fascism, a group that had a large communist membership. He saw no reason not to co-operate with communists, who shared with the CCFers the desire to end capitalism, and also was active in another organization with communist ties, the Canadian Youth Congress. In 1936, he traveled as a CYC delegate to an international youth conference in Geneva.

Tommy's own positions weren't always what one would expect. For example, he opposed a Liberal plan to issue banknotes with both English and French words on them, an early gesture toward bilingualism, because he feared they would spark a backlash of bigotry in the West. The government should leave "well enough alone, by letting sleeping dogs lie," he told Parliament.

More often, though, Tommy was "on the side of the angels," prodding the Liberals to do more for the West, for farmers, for poor people, and to oppose fascism.

Years later, journalist Bruce Hutchison summed up Tommy's eight-year stint in Ottawa this way: "He fought as he had fought in the amateur boxing ring... with sudden, quick punches, rapid footwork, and, above all, with courage. He did not make himself popular in Parliament, but he made himself heard, and, at times, he could penetrate even the rhinoceros skin of the government."

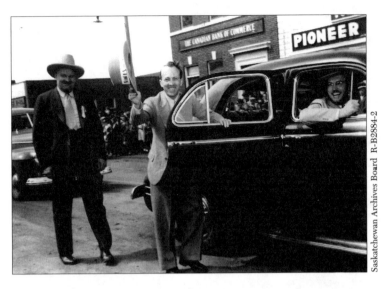

Tommy Douglas mainstreeting after – his criticism of government war policies having made him a national figure – he switches to provincial politics. "My friends, watch out for the little fellow with an idea."

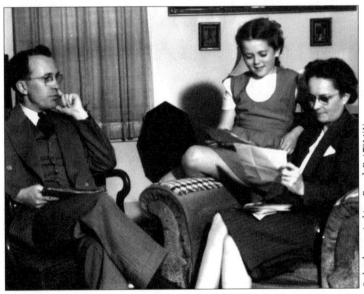

Ten-year-old Shirley Douglas sits with her parents on the night the CCF wins the 1944 election and her father becomes Premier of Saskatchewan.

7

Victory in Saskatchewan

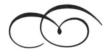

June 15, 1944, election night in Saskatchewan. In Tommy Douglas's committee rooms at the Weyburn Legion Hall, young Tom McLeod, a protégé of Tommy's, is manning the phones.

Ten-year-old Shirley, her hair in pigtails, comes running in. "Is my father the premier yet?" she asks breathlessly.

"Not yet," McLeod replies, smiling. He picks up another phone.

The smell of victory is in the air. In Europe, Allied forces are fighting their way up from the beaches of Normandy, where they landed nine days ago, and there's a sense that the war will soon be over. In Saskatchewan, people can taste better times.

Party workers have set up an elaborate provincewide telephone network, with all calls leading to the Weyburn committee rooms. By 9:00 p.m., it's clear Tommy's won his own riding – a victory made especially sweet because it's the same provincial riding he was beaten in ten years earlier, in his first campaign.

"Is my father premier yet?" Shirley wants to know.

"Pretty soon," McLeod tells her. "Pretty soon." The phone is ringing again.

By 10:00 p.m., Shirley doesn't have to ask. News of riding victories are pouring in from all over the province: forty-seven out of fifty-two seats won by the Co-operative Commonwealth Federation (CCF). Before the night is over, Shirley watches as her father is carried on the shoulders of his supporters down Main Street.

∞

"In the dark days of the Depression," Tommy remembered, "I used to ask the minister of finance why the government couldn't get industry moving again, develop our resources, provide jobs for the unemployed, and his answer to me was, 'Young man, money doesn't grow on gooseberry bushes.'...Well, then came the war, and they found the bush!"

When Britain declared war on Germany in September, 1939, Canada quickly followed suit. MP Tommy Douglas immediately enlisted and rushed home to Weyburn to join the South Saskatchewan Regiment. After the long Depression, there were plenty of men with no jobs or families who were eager to fight, and "the boys were coming off the boxcars and into the recruiting stations," he said.

He joined as a corporal but was soon commissioned as an officer, rising to captain. Tommy declined an offer to be a chaplain, and his wartime experience was confined to training others; he never was sent overseas, and his battles were staged in the halls of Parliament.

He did come close to seeing action, though – and to losing his life.

In October 1941, two Canadian units, the Royal Rifles of Quebec and the Winnipeg Grenadiers, were sent to reinforce the British garrison at Hong Kong. Tommy was one of six officers in a group of a hundred from Saskatchewan who were transferred to the Grenadiers. He was all set to ship out, but at the last minute he was turned down because of concern over his old leg injury, although, ironically, the leg was causing him no problem at the time.

Within weeks of their arrival, Hong Kong was invaded by the Japanese, who caught the garrison unprepared. Many of the Canadians were killed; those who survived spent the rest of the war in prison camps. Tommy's national profile rose after he became a vocal critic of the government in the furor that followed the fall of Hong Kong. A government inquiry was established after charges that the Canadian troops had not been properly trained or equipped, and Tommy's speech on the issue in the House was so eloquent it was published in full in the next day's *Globe and Mail*.

Tommy caustic attack on the Hong Kong fiasco was criticized by some as unpatriotic, a charge he shrugged off in characteristic fashion: "If there was inefficiency and incompetence at Hong Kong, there was no point in trying to keep it from the Japanese. They knew all about it."

Tommy had been a critic of government war policies since the summer of 1936, when, while on a trip to Europe, he saw Nazis marching in the streets of Germany and heard tales of unionists sent to prison camps. "I recognized then that if you came to a choice between losing freedom of speech, religion, association, thought...and resorting to force, you'd use force," he said. This put him at odds with both Woodsworth and Coldwell, committed pacifists. It also created a rift between Tommy and his communist associates when, after the Hitler-Stalin non-aggression treaty in 1939, they changed their anti-fascist rhetoric to opposition to war with Germany. Tommy wrote a magazine article condemning Canadian communists for their turnaround that was headlined "I Am Disgusted."

Canada's declaration of war was traumatic for the small CCF caucus because Woodsworth, loyal to his pacifist ideals, wouldn't go along. In the end, the leader handed the party reins to Coldwell and spoke against the war as an individual while Tommy and the others voted for Canada to support the war effort, though they stopped short at sending troops. M.J., who had been a strong supporter of the party's previous policy of neutrality, called it the most difficult decision of his life.

Tommy also was active in a failed CCF campaign to limit war profiteering. "Let there be no conscription of men without a conscription of wealth," he argued.

"Let there be some equality in sacrifice." The Mackenzie King government accepted the CCF proposal – a limit of 5 per cent on war-related profits – but quickly dropped it when industry refused to go along. "It was scandalous," Tommy said. "The arms manufacturers actually went on strike. If the workers, or the soldiers, had taken such a position, think of the outcry."

Almost immediately after the onset of war, though, he was fighting another election, which King called for March 1940 and won with a huge majority. The Weyburn campaign, waged through a cold, snowy winter, was unremarkable, and Tommy, pitted only against a Liberal candidate, won by almost a thousand votes. The CCF improved its fortunes too: it elected eight members, five of them from Saskatchewan, making the province the heart of the national party.

One dark spot on the CCF's wartime record was its support, along with other parties, of the government's treatment of Japanese Canadians; even Tommy Douglas remained mostly silent as thousands of West Coast Japanese were rounded up and sent to prison camps, their property seized and sold at auction.

Between his duties in Parliament and the army, and with the easing of Depression conditions that had previously captured so much of his attention, Tommy's energies were focused heavily on the war for the next few years. With Coldwell now the national leader, Tommy was his unofficial lieutenant, but this stage of his life was about to end.

Saskatchewan was calling.

∽

In fact, Tommy had never really given up his interest in provincial politics. All through his years in Parliament, he remained active in the Saskatchewan CCF. He formed a close working relationship with George Williams, the man who had tried so hard to have him expelled from the party for his arrangement with Social Credit. Williams, who became party leader when Coldwell went to Ottawa in 1935, was also party president and chairman of the council that oversaw the party's operations. Despite this iron grip, or perhaps because of it, the party's fortunes were declining. It emerged from a 1938 provincial election with only eleven seats, double what it had won in 1934, but not nearly as many as had been expected – "a terrible schmozzle," as Tommy wryly put it. The CCF was the Official Opposition in Regina, but there was discontent within the party's leadership.

There was also discontent with Williams from Ottawa, where Coldwell became national CCF leader soon after the onset of war. M.J. began to suggest to Tommy that his most valuable contribution to the party might lie back home in Saskatchewan.

Tommy tended to agree that Williams's "one-man show" had become more of a problem than a strength. "It was apparent something had to be done," he said. If not, "there was a growing feeling that we were doomed."

But Tommy, who, before war broke out, had been thinking of not running for Parliament again and resuming his Ph.D. studies, wasn't all that keen on returning to the Saskatchewan fray. "What influenced me really," he recalled, "was that farmers came to me

and said, 'A lot of us are losing our farms. The prices
we're getting aren't adequate to pay off the huge accu-
mulation of debt. Farms are being foreclosed, there are
evictions, machinery is being repossessed. If you can't
do anything else but get us some type of debt adjust-
ment, some security.... You can make speeches in
Ottawa, but you can do at least this much because we
can form a government here.'"

It was a seductive argument.

Not everybody in the Saskatchewan wing of the
party's leadership thought Tommy was the man to fill
Williams's shoes, though. Carlyle King, a University of
Saskatchewan English professor whose pacifism had
led to bruising disagreements with Williams, dismissed
Tommy too, calling him "practically an imperialist."
King said, "My guess is that Douglas will not be with us
long, for which we can be truly thankful." Before long,
though, he switched gears and became a strong supporter.

Williams himself brought the issue to a head by
joining the army and going overseas. At the provincial
convention in July 1941, Tommy won the party presidency. Because Williams had been leader as well as
president, Tommy assumed he'd inherited that job as
well, but there was some resistance, and the leadership
stayed up for grabs until another convention, early in
1942, when Tommy was confirmed. Clarence Fines, a
Regina alderman who had been Coldwell's assistant
principal, became president of the party. John
Brockelbank, an MLA who had been temporary leader
after Williams's departure and who was loyal to Williams,
was hand-picked by Tommy to be vice-president.

Any acrimony that may have existed in the wake of Tommy's winning the leadership quickly dissolved. Tommy was just too much of a charmer, too skilled a "people person," to make enemies; he quickly mended fences and delegated authority. As Brockelbank, a potential rival, saw it: "Tommy was a diplomat, George wasn't."

Tommy himself put it this way: "My main job was to get everybody working together." The party, he said, "was like a symphony orchestra; my part was to beat the time and keep everybody playing on the same score."

∞

It was a great time to be a socialist in Canada. The CCF's popularity was soaring, all across the country. The party had become Official Opposition in British Columbia and Ontario, joining Saskatchewan, and now Tommy set his sights on forming government.

The Liberal machine of Jimmy Gardiner had still enjoyed a hold over voters in 1938, when so many were on relief and were told in no uncertain terms: "Vote Liberal or be kicked off the rolls."

"It was a terrible thing to watch," Tommy said. "It was a complete negation of democracy."

But now, people were unafraid to vote their own minds. Worse still for the Saskatchewan Liberals, the government, under Premier William Patterson, Gardiner's hand-picked successor, was tired and out of ideas. An election should have been called for 1942, or 1943 at the latest, but Patterson clung to power and postponed it to June 1944. He cited the need for stability during the war but the delay further irritated voters.

It also worked to the CCF's advantage, giving Tommy more time to organize the party and prepare for the campaign. If Patterson "had called the election in '42 or '43, we would have had a close call," he said later. "By the end of '43, the tide had turned and nothing could save him."

A nationwide attack on the CCF, led by Bay Street bankers and industrialists and joined by the nation's newspapers, claimed that socialists were just communists in sheep's clothing, that CCF governments would confiscate property, insurance policies, and bank accounts. After the Saskatchewan election was called, the Liberals added to the scare list claims that the CCF would close both the churches and the beer parlours. Tommy and his party were characterized both as communists and nazis – quite a feat. "The attacks became more hysterical with every passing day," Tommy remembered.

The Liberal campaign sank to a new low with a pathetic slogan used on posters and newspaper ads: "Please Give Us Another Chance."

Saskatchewan's newspapers did everything they could to stop Tommy's momentum; they even suppressed a Gallop Poll survey that predicted a CCF victory and ran their own poll that showed the Liberals ahead. *The Regina Leader Post* predicted Tommy Douglas as premier would usher in a "stultifying dictatorial system."

Tommy and the party fought back with a simple platform and a candidates' school, to ensure everyone running on the CCF ticket understood it. Tommy himself and David Lewis from the Ottawa office were among the instructors. Tommy's advice: "You stand up, you speak up, you shut up." The platform called for a law ensuring farm security, support for co-ops, a shakeup of public schools, the beginnings of a system of Crown corporations and the first steps toward socialized health care.

The CCF's most powerful weapon, though, was Tommy himself. He was a tireless, eager campaigner with a magic voice and a seemingly magic touch.

Long before the word "charisma" had been applied to politicians, Tommy had it, and long before television made it easy for a politician to have a provincewide presence, Tommy earned it.

Grace MacInnis, Woodsworth's daughter, said Tommy became "the living symbol" of the better future the party promised Saskatchewan. Grant MacNeil, a CCF member of Parliament from Vancouver, said Tommy was the key to the party's election hopes: "He was head and shoulders above everyone out there."

Stanley Knowles, Tommy's old friend from Brandon College who had joined him in Parliament, agreed. "Fines couldn't have done it. No one else on the scene could have. Saskatchewan was ripe for the CCF in 1944, but would they have won it with George Williams? I don't think so."

Tommy, Knowles said, "was the man."

What he was for certain was a man continually on the go. He was on the road from dawn to after dark, attending meeting after meeting, rally after rally, picnic after picnic. He preferred to ad lib and rarely wrote out his speeches, but wartime regulations that required anything for broadcast to be viewed by a censor forced him to sit down and write his talks for the radio.

"I wrote a lot of broadcasts at night until two or three o'clock in the morning in the hotels after a meeting was over," he recalled. "Many times, I'd ride half the night, get a few hours sleep, write a broadcast, record it, and then get on the road again."

It was a gruelling schedule but Tommy seemed to thrive on it. "This is the politician's heaviest cross," he said, half complaining, half joking. "He needs sleep, not food, and everyone wants to feed him rather than let him sleep."

In all his talks, Tommy hammered away at his two favourite topics: health care and the plight of the farmer.

He promised steps to diversify the economy, now so completely dependent on wheat, and to face down the eastern bankers so eager to throw western farmers off their land. Saskatchewan would have "farm security legislation on the statute books before the snow fell," he pledged.

And he promised to do something about a health care situation that sent 65 per cent of Canadians into debt to pay for surgery.

But he was realistic, cautioning his listeners not to expect "an entire new society. Nobody can do that in one province." In the Canadian system, only the federal government has powers over money, tariffs, freight rates, and other issues vital to Saskatchewan, and Tommy didn't want the CCF "to get one vote in this election by saying they are going to do things they cannot constitutionally do," as Social Credit had in Alberta.

Everywhere he went, Tommy charmed and won over the voters, not with empty talk or inflated promises, but with a hard-headed, realistic appraisal of their situation and with parables like those Jesus told – spiced with a sense of humour all his own.

One favourite he told over and over again began with his recollection of visiting a farm and getting stuck helping with the chores. Turning the handle on the cream separator, he began to think how much the old-fashioned machine resembled the capitalistic system. "There were the farmers pouring in good fresh milk. There were the city workers, turning the handle. And out of two spouts came blue milk for the workers and farmers, cream for the guys who owned the machine. When those guys got a bellyache from too much rich cream, they held up a hand and said, 'Stop! Hold it! No more milk. This is a Depression!'"

The story he liked to tell best – and the one people most loved to hear – was about Mouseland, where the cats were in power. Every four years, the mice would elect one group of cats or another. The cats were smart, and they passed good laws – for cats. "But, oh, they were hard on the mice," Tommy would say, rolling his eyes. Under the black cats, conditions were terrible for the mice, so after four years they threw them out and gave power to the white cats. But the white cats were even hungrier and crueler, so in the next election the black cats were given another chance. On and on it went, and the mice always got the short end of the stick.

Until one day, when one mouse had a bright idea: "Say," he said, "why don't we elect *mice*?"

The cats, and even some of the mice, called him a radical, a commie, a nazi rat, but the other mice began to talk about the idea, and the idea spread.

"My friends," Tommy would finish, with a wink, "watch out for the little fellow with an idea."

On election night, it seemed the mice of Saskatchewan had gotten the idea. As Tommy watched the results come in, he knew the fight had really only begun. "I had no illusions that I was starting on a honeymoon," he said. "I kept remembering what the farmers had said. 'If you can just save our farms, if you can just do that much.'"

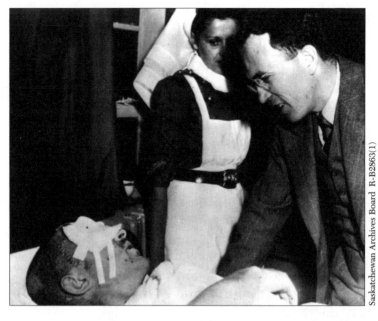

In March 1945 Tommy visits Saskatchewan troops in Europe
after sailing on a troop ship through the submarine-infested
waters of the North Atlantic.

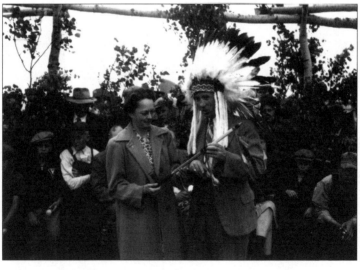

Irma Douglas inspects her husband's regalia after he is made
Chief Red Eagle (*We-a-ga-sha*) by the Assiniboine
Indian Band at Carlyle Lake.

8

Tommy Douglas in Power

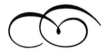

A lovely autumn evening in Sturgis, Saskatchewan, 1944. The crop has been harvested and prices are decent. The war looks to be over soon, the boys coming home. And there's that new government in Regina, making all sorts of wild promises.

Tommy Douglas, the new premier, is talking at a meeting at the old schoolhouse. Light is fading and the kerosene lanterns are lit. The lanterns, he claims, can soon be thrown away!

"We're going to harness the Churchill River in the north and mine coal at Estevan, and run an electrical grid over all of Saskatchewan," the premier says excitedly.

A big, burly man at the back of the room laughs. "Mr. Douglas, you're a dreamer."

Tommy just smiles.

A few years later, he's in Sturgis again, this time to open a new school, a centrally heated school with plumbing, and lit by electricity. A man approaches him. "Excuse me, Mr. Douglas, do you remember me?"

"You look familiar, but I don't remember meeting you," Tommy confesses.

"It was a meeting you held in that little school-house," the man says, with a little embarrassment, "and there was a man at the back who got up and said you were a dreamer. That was me. I didn't think you could do it."

∞

Newspapers across North America declared that Tommy Douglas had established "a beachhead of socialism on a continent of capitalism."

In Saskatchewan, the mood was buoyant, even jubilant, among supporters of the new government, suspicious, even fearful, among those who had voted against the CCF.

And the province itself was virtually bankrupt. It had been unable to borrow money on the open market since 1932, and found itself now facing a hostile business community, a hostile press, and a hostile federal government.

Whatever Saskatchewan was going to do to reform its systems, to improve the conditions of its people, and forge progressive new programs, Tommy knew, it would have to do on its own.

The idea of socialism, Tommy always said, is ridiculously easy. It means spreading the wealth so that no one has more than he needs, and no one else goes wanting – to each according to his need, from each according to his ability to pay. The practice of socialism, he was soon to discover, isn't so easy. Those who have, don't want to give it up, and the institutions of a capitalistic, free-enterprise society, driven by market forces, resist change. Tommy Douglas and the CCF came to power in Saskatchewan promising socialism, and they did begin to make moves in that direction, but over fifty years later it's still open to debate how successful they were.

Tommy was a committed socialist who was also committed to the principles of democracy. He understood that power involved a delicate balancing act: satisfying your supporters, mollifying your foes, not spooking the onlooking crowd by moving too fast. The philosophy of gradualism became his watchword, persuasion – gentle, and spiced with humour – his most effective tool. He was fond of quoting an old Scottish adage: "If you canna see the bottom, dinna wade far oot."

The key to turning socialistic theory into practice, Tommy was certain, was a planned economy.

But who does the planning?

The government that took power in Regina in 1944 was a creature not just of a party – the CCF – but of a progressive, socialistic movement. Who was it accountable to? The party? The socialist cause? Or the people of Saskatchewan at large?

Two days after he was sworn in, Tommy went on the radio to warn mortgage companies against foreclosing on any more farms. In that same broadcast, he assured Saskatchewan that he was the premier of all the people, not just the ones who voted for him, and not just members of his party.

There was an enormous amount of work to do, and many in Saskatchewan and the rest of the country sat back with skeptical smirks on their faces and waited for the new premier to stumble and fall.

Sometimes he did stumble. Mostly, though, he was on the mark, and as one journalist put it, Premier Tommy Douglas "presided over the province's leap into the twentieth century."

Tommy "made first class citizens out of us in Saskatchewan," said Roy Borrowman, who was recruited by the premier fresh out of the army into the civil service. "Before that time, we always looked upon the East and said, 'There's where it is. There's where the money is, there's where the opportunities are. We don't have much chance in Saskatchewan.' After Tommy came...we could hold our heads up and say, 'We're just as good as anyone. We can take our place with anybody.'"

Within its first year in office, the government Tommy led achieved many of the promises of its election platform. The first tentative steps toward medicare were taken, and there were free textbooks in the schools; a government automobile insurance company was created (the first of its kind in the world), and a law passed to protect debt-ridden farmers. He also began to overhaul the civil service, invited government workers to form unions – years ahead of other provinces – and passed the most advanced labour code in the country, which guaranteed workers the right to organize and brought in the closed shop and automatic dues checkoff. Another law provided for two weeks paid holiday, putting Saskatchewan workers way ahead of their fellows in other provinces.

One Toronto newspaper said Saskatchewan had established Canada's "socialist guinea pig government." Another grudgingly declared the CCF regime "the flagship of social change for all of Canada."

∞

The day after the election, Tom McLeod went to call on the premier-in-waiting.

"How would you like to work for the new government?" Tommy asked.

McLeod had been a member of the boys' club Tommy organized at Calvary Baptist Church and he'd been devoted to the older man ever since. Like Tommy, he went to Brandon College, then went on to get a doctorate in economics at Indiana and was back at Brandon teaching. He'd spent the summer in Weyburn, working on Tommy's campaign. "I guess so," he stammered.

"That's fortunate," Tommy said. "I've already wired your resignation to the college."

McLeod became economic adviser to cabinet and helped Tommy recruit a small army of bright people, some of them socialists, others only sympathetic to the cause. The woman Tommy picked to be his personal secretary, Eleanor McKinnon, was the daughter of a Calvary Baptist deacon and prominent Liberal. She was a Brandon College graduate and had worked as secretary to the superintendent of the Weyburn mental hospital. The transition to the premier's office in the legislature building in Regina, where madness often seemed to rule, may have been an easy one for her. At any rate, she soon became the calm in the centre of the storm, keeping Tommy on track, sorting through the mountains of mail that began to flood in, and keeping away the nutcases. She would remain at Tommy's side, in Regina and Ottawa, for the next forty-two years.

Clarence Fines, the Regina schoolteacher who'd become the organizational genius for the Saskatchewan CCF, was Tommy's right hand as provincial treasurer and deputy premier.

In the CCF contingent elected, six were union members, mostly railroaders; a few were teachers, but the majority were farmers. Tommy presided over a rag-tag cabinet of untried ministers like a ringmaster at a three-ring circus. "The cabinet was a good cross-section of people," Fines said. "Average people with a lot of enthusiasm and devotion. We had a vision; that made the difference." Tom McLeod said Tommy's "leadership was beyond dispute. No challengers. No questioners." In his dealing with people, Tommy was "the smoothest customer I ever saw," Fines said.

When ministers or other government officials flagged, the watchword would be: "Go and hear Tommy and get your batteries re-charged."

One of the new premier's first acts was to increase the size of cabinet from nine to twelve, adding departments of labour, co-operatives, and social welfare. To deflect criticism of free spending, he cut salaries for ministers from $7,000 to $5,000, with his own pay at

$6,500. Among those in that first cabinet, along with Fines, were Woodrow Lloyd, a young teacher and head of the provincial teachers' union, who became education minister, and John Brockelbank, who had run against Tommy for the party leadership a few years earlier and who now became minister of municipal affairs. Although they'd once been seriously at odds, Tommy had encouraged George Williams to run, and he'd won the seat for Wadena as an absentee candidate while still in Europe with the army. He was picked to be agriculture minister but, before he could take up his duties, suffered a stroke and died soon afterward.

There were no women in cabinet – in fact, there was only one woman, Beatrice Trew from Maple Creek, in the CCF caucus during the first term.

Tommy and his team were able to move quickly on their program because they had done their homework and were ready to swing into action as soon as they took office.

But at the same time, Premier Douglas looked more and more to experts, many of them recruited from outside the province, for ideas and the ability to put them into motion. For example, a team of health care experts, including several from the U.S., quickly came up with plans for what would eventually become the medicare program.

Loyal CCFers became incensed that some of these experts weren't even socialists. But, as Tommy cautioned his critics, "it's easier to make a socialist out of an engineer than it is to make an engineer out of a socialist."

∞

The CCF may have been the overwhelming choice of the people, but that didn't stop the Liberals from sniping at their heels. Reduced to a rump of only five members in the legislature, they still did everything they could to make things rough for the new boys in power.

The government was sworn in on July 10, 1944, by Lieutenant-Governor Archibald P. McNab. Hundreds of people attended the ceremony at the magnificent black-domed Tyndall stone Legislative Building, with its marble floors and pillars and sweeping grand staircase. It was the first time the ceremony had ever been held in public. Among them was Tommy's proud mother, Anne, decked out in a formal gown and large hat and given a seat of honour on the floor of the legislative chamber.

But when Tommy and his cabinet members went off to their new offices, they found all the filing cabinets had been stripped bare, an act of vandalism by the sour-grapes former government.

Tommy, who took the health portfolio as well as the premier's duties for himself, happened to run into the former Liberal health minister, Dr. John Uhrich, soon after the election, and he asked Uhrich if he had any advice.

"You made all the promises, you know all the answers, so you go ahead and see how you make out," Uhrich snapped back.

One Liberal MLA was evicted from the legislative assembly that first session after calling Tommy "a stinking skunk."

Most of his critics were more civil. And the new premier was a genius at calming down people opposed to his changes, at winning at least some of them over.

Meeting with a group of suspicious doctors, he explained why he'd taken the health portfolio himself: "It's a pity no doctors ran. I think we should have more doctors in the legislature; I hope some of you will run on future occasions. But you'll have to put up with me, and there is a place for laymen in the administration of health services."

Then he told them the story of his childhood bout with osteomyelitis, how he would have lost his leg but for the charity of one interested doctor.

Another time, he came out of the legislature to talk to a crowd of about a thousand hissing and booing truckers angry over a hefty increase in licence fees. Tommy waited, calmly smiling, until the noise tapered off, then he told them how much he sympathized with them, trying to make a living on Saskatchewan's corrugated, pothole-filled roads, the worst in the country. He told them how the road improvements the government was planning would help them out, and about the cheap insurance he was going to bring in. And, Tommy being Tommy, he had them laughing at his jokes and applauding.

Later, driving home, a few of the truckers were talking about what a great guy the premier was. "Yeah, but what about the licences we came here to squawk about?" one of them suddenly asked. "The little son-of-a-gun never even mentioned them."

∞

When the CCF took power, Saskatchewan was $178 million in debt, about the equivalent today of $17 billion! Clarence Fines earmarked 10 per cent of each year's budget to pay off the debt. By the time they left office twenty years later, it was virtually gone.

The CCF under Tommy and Fines avoided further debt by setting money aside in a "sugar bowl" account to pay for new schools, hospitals, roads, and government buildings. They didn't get built until there was sufficient money available.

Fines' first budget was about $40 million. (Today, the Saskatchewan budget is close to $6 billion, about 150 times greater.)

Like good Saskatchewan farmers, what they couldn't afford to buy, they scrounged, borrowed, or re-used. Millions of dollars worth of army surplus equipment was grabbed up at six to eight cents on the dollar. Air force hangers became community skating rinks, and little towns suddenly boasted fire engines bought for a song. Thousands of Saskatchewan farms got new paint jobs, with veterans manning surplus spraying rigs.

Tommy opened the doors of the legislature as they never had been before, making debates available in printed form and on instantly popular live radio broadcasts, the first in Canada. As a result, the daily doings of the government became dinner table and coffee shop chatter all across the province. And with good reason. What the government down in Regina was doing was having sweeping effects on everybody in Saskatchewan.

∞

Tommy Douglas was the odd man out when, in the summer of 1945, he attended a federal-provincial conference to plan a new relationship for the postwar era. Mackenzie King, fearing the CCF on his left, had developed a grand design that included social insurance, unemployment insurance, and tax sharing. Tommy, a firm believer in a strong central government, supported the plan, but the other premiers, fearing a loss of their own power, were all opposed, and the plan foundered.

But usually Saskatchewan's fights were with the federal government, not other provinces.

The most dramatic was the long struggle over the farm debt situation.

As promised, a law protecting farmers from creditors was among the very first passed by the legislature in the fall of 1944. The Farm Security Act prevented banks and mortgage companies from foreclosing on the home quarter – that part of a farm that contains the farmer's house and outbuildings – and suspended payments in years of crop failures, when farmers just couldn't pay. That was bad enough for the mortgage holders to swallow but they really choked on another provision, which wiped out interest in the bad years as well. Tommy's theory was that the banks profited when the farmers did, so they should be prepared to take the same risks.

The moneylenders predictably went running to Ottawa, and King threatened to disallow the law, a rarely used provision under the constitution. That federal power had been successfully used to pull the teeth out of Social Credit's more radical programs in Alberta. Now, Liberals who had warned the CCF would steal people's homes were threatening to give legal comfort to banks, which were doing just that.

Tommy got on the radio to rouse the population: "We have just finished a war which was fought, we were told, for the preservation of democratic institutions. It would appear that the war is not finished. We have simply moved the battlefields from the banks of the Rhine to the prairies of Saskatchewan."

Tommy said if the law was disallowed, his government would take other measures to protect farmers. He would not "retreat one single inch," he vowed. And he urged his listeners to join him in the struggle: "We are prepared to lead that fight if you are prepared to follow us into battle."

The result was a deluge of letters to Ottawa and mass rallies throughout the province to denounce the federal plan.

Mackenzie King's government backed down on disallowing the law, but it did challenge in the courts the clause that cancelled interest in bad years. The case wound its way through the courts over the next few years, going all the way to the Supreme Court of Canada, which ruled the Saskatchewan government didn't have the power to rob the moneylenders of their interest. The Privy Council of England – which under the British North America Act, the Canadian constitution of the day, had final say – agreed.

The CCF fought back with another law that also was eventually defeated in the courts in 1958. In the meantime, though, Saskatchewan farmers had some protection.

Another area of friction with the federal government was the Indians of Saskatchewan.

Tommy took an interest in native affairs, although the federal government had clear responsibility for Indians. He had a friendly relationship with the Indian band at Carlyle Lake, where the Douglas family had a summer cottage, and soon after becoming premier he was given an Assiniboine name, *We-a-ga-sha*, or Chief Red Eagle. Seeing the impoverished state of the then fourteen thousand status Indians on the province's sixty-one reserves, he brought their chiefs together and helped them form the Union of Saskatchewan Indians, the first such organization in the province, to negotiate with Ottawa as a single voice.

Ottawa was not amused.

Indians were also granted the vote in Saskatchewan for the first time – ironically, the first time they had a chance to use it, they voted heavily against the CCF – and were given the dubious right to buy alcohol, even though drunkenness was a serious problem among native people. Tommy, who rarely drank himself, took a philosophical approach: "If liquor is bad for us, it is bad for the Indian. But there has to be the same law for all." More importantly, he attempted for years to persuade Ottawa to transfer responsibility for the neglected Indians in Saskatchewan to the province, along with appropriate financial compensation, but got nowhere. Efforts to assist Métis communities in Saskatchewan were somewhat more successful, since they fell under provincial jurisdiction.

One of the longest running arguments with Ottawa was over damming the South Saskatchewan River. The CCF wanted a dam, and the reservoir it would create, as a water source for irrigation and drinking, as well as for recreation. In fact, people had been talking about the possibility for years. But former premier Jimmy Gardiner, now agriculture minister in Mackenzie King's government, began making promises in 1944, soon after the CCF came to power in Saskatchewan. Unfortunately, King himself was disinterested, and his successor, Louis St. Laurent, had no interest at all. Through a decade of negotiations, Tommy got nowhere and often felt he was beating his head against a stone wall.

On one visit to Ottawa, he met with St. Laurent and Gardiner and, as the prime minister made it clear he wouldn't contribute a penny to the project, his minister from Saskatchewan sat silent as a freshwater clam. But as Tommy was leaving, Gardiner caught up with him in the hallway. "Now don't you pay any attention to that," he blustered. "He doesn't mean what he says. Why don't we just go into my office and talk about it?"

An exasperated Tommy lost his temper. "You go to hell," he snapped. "I don't want to discuss this with you at all."

The dam finally won approval in 1958 when the Conservatives, under John Diefenbaker, another Saskatchewan boy, came to national power, but it wasn't completed and officially opened, by Liberal Prime Minister Lester Pearson, until 1967, twenty-three years after Gardiner's first promises. In an ironic political hat trick, the dam was named for Gardiner, the lake for Diefenbaker, and the provincial park surrounding them for Douglas.

Through it all, Tommy kept the faith.

One night in the legislature, a young opposition member scolded him, saying it was too bad a Baptist minister had turned into a socialist premier. Tommy could only smile. "It's true that eighteen years ago I dedicated myself to serve the Kingdom of God," he said, "and if I didn't believe I was still doing that, I would not be standing here today."

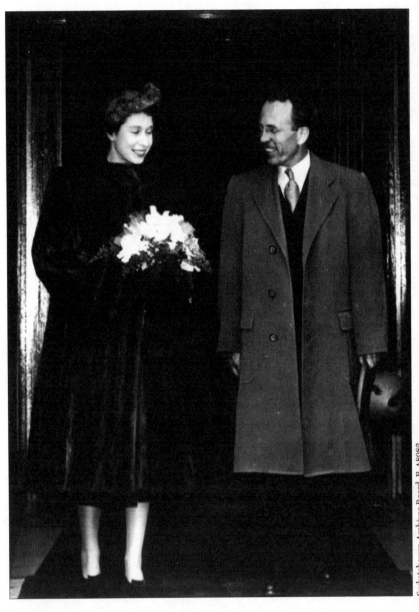

"A dreamer and a humanitarian, incorruptible, genuine and intellectually honest," the socialist premier of Saskatchewan greets Princess Elizabeth in 1951.

9

A First-Rate Leader

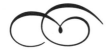

A story Tommy liked to tell while campaigning:
A politician on the hustings is delighted one day
when he comes across an old friend. Here, he's certain,
is a vote he can count on. But the old friend soon
reveals that he's undecided.

"What? How can you say that?" asks the astonished
candidate. "When we were boys together, we went skating and you fell through the ice and I pulled you out."

The old friend nods his head.

"When you wanted to get married," the politician
continues, "I loaned you two hundred dollars."

Again, a nod of the head.

"When your house burned down, I signed a note
for you at the bank."

"Yes, yes," the friend agrees. "I remember."

" And when your child needed an operation, I loaned you the money you needed. Isn't that so?" the politician demands.

"That's all true," the old friend replies. "But what have you done for me lately?"

∽

The face of the Saskatchewan countryside changed drastically during the two decades the CCF was in power. Tommy was constantly "doing something lately." Thousands of miles of roads and highways were paved – in 1944, there were only 138 miles (222 km) of black-top in the province – and electricity was brought to most farmyards. Health and education improved; incomes rose, and thousands of people enjoyed a sense of security they'd only dreamed of before.

The government also turned its attention to quality of life matters, establishing a provincial archives and the Saskatchewan Arts Board, the first such agency in North America, to foster the arts in the province. Liquor laws were relaxed, allowing women to join men in beer parlours and cocktail lounges, and drinks to be served in restaurants. The network of provincial and regional parks was expanded. The first small claims court in North America was established. A Bill of Rights, prohibiting discrimination based on race, colour, or religion, was adopted in 1946, years ahead of other provinces and the federal government. As soon as the war ended, Tommy invited uprooted and interned Canadian Japanese to resettle in

Saskatchewan, the only premier to put out the welcome mat.

Most of these things cost money.

While other issues often got more attention from the public and the press, much of the effort of the government was directed at economic matters. It was vital to Saskatchewan's interests to diversify and grow the economy, Tommy argued, so it wouldn't be so dependent on wheat.

Two key instruments of that growth were co-operatives (like the already active Saskatchewan Wheat Pool) and Crown (government-owned) corporations.

What he had in mind, Tommy said, was "a mixed economy combining public ownership, co-operative ownership, and private ownership."

Saskatchewan already had power and telephone Crowns, which were now aggressively expanded, and the government jumped into the insurance business with both feet. On a smaller scale, the CCF got into transportation, taking over money-losing bus lines and even starting a northern airline service. Before long, there was a government-owned printing plant, box factory, tannery, woollen mill, even a shoe factory. Early in its first term, the CCF backed a scheme to convert agricultural produce into plastics, quietly dropping it later. For a while, the government was even behind a project that saw herds of wild horses running loose in southwestern Saskatchewan ranch country rounded up and slaughtered for sale to meat-hungry postwar Europe. That venture actually was a success, but most of these smaller projects lost money and were abandoned after a while.

But the Crowns were never intended to be more than a stimulus to the larger, mostly privately owned, economy. "The CCF does not want to own everything," Tommy declared. "The only freedom we were taking away was the freedom to exploit someone else." And when Tommy was reminded on the floor of the legislature, by one of his own MLAs, that the Regina Manifesto had called for an end to capitalism, the premier replied his government would encourage private business "wherever it did not interfere with the welfare of the people." Capitalism as it had been known prior to the Depression was gone, Tommy was convinced. In fact, the government did everything it could to encourage private investment and was wildly successful. Despite its bad rap in the eastern-dominated press and throughout the business world, individual businesses found plenty to like in Saskatchewan, and, from 1948 to 1960, the province had the highest rate of growth in the country, fuelled to a large extent by discoveries of oil, natural gas, potash, and uranium. The CCF government had a hand in the development of all of these industries, and also brought steel to the province.

Along the way, Saskatchewan ironically became, as *The Globe and Mail* pointed out, "the biggest booster of free enterprise on the prairies."

Saskatchewan was transformed, but Tommy always felt as if one hand was tied behind his back. There was only so much a provincial government could do, as long as the real reins of power lay in Ottawa, and as Tommy's seventeen years as premier entered its final phase, he began thinking again of entering the national arena. "No one," he said, "can build an island of social-ism in a sea of capitalism."

∞

Tommy proved to be a master communicator as much in power as on the campaign trail. Through an endless series of speeches, radio broadcasts, newspaper and magazine articles, and literally thousands of letters, which he dictated to his secretary, Eleanor McKinnon, he kept up a steady dialogue with the people of Saskatchewan and, to a lesser extent, of Canada.

In a series of Sunday evening radio "fireside chats," Tommy avoided politics, and instead enter-tained his listeners with recitations from Burns, Kipling, Longfellow, and of course, the Bible, just as he had as a boy and young man.

The idea of a professional speechwriter would have made Tommy laugh, and he usually got exasper-ated when his aides did attempt to pen something for him, invariably finding their efforts too filled with jar-gon and "bureaucratese." Once, to illustrate his point, he produced a letter from a voter who complained about the provincial power corporation's intrusions onto his land. In the middle of the letter was this suc-cinct line: "Some bugger bust my fence."

"There it is," Tommy said triumphantly, about to deliver a grammar lesson: "Subject, 'bugger'; verb, 'bust'; object, 'fence'. Why can't you fellows write like that?"

∞

As premier and party leader, Tommy put in long days and, except for summer holidays, always spent with the family at their cottage at Carlyle Lake, he rarely took a break.

His day began with a breakfast of orange juice, oatmeal, toast, and coffee with Irma and the girls (a second daughter, Joan, was adopted in 1940). Then he would snack on raisin pie – he had a passion for the stuff – and coffee through the day, until an ulcer he'd picked up a few years earlier flared up again. He switched to sipping milk and had a lunch of tomato juice, poached egg on toast, and prunes at the legislature cafeteria, standing in line with everyone else. If he knew he'd be out in the afternoon and likely to be late for supper, he'd often fortify himself with a double milkshake with a raw egg in it.

He was not quite forty when he was elected, and would be fifty-seven when he left the premier's job, still in fighting trim, carrying 145 pounds (65.8 kg) on his wiry five-foot, six-inch (1.68-metre) frame. His light brown curly hair was receding from his high forehead, and a pair of wire-rimmed glasses perched on his small pug nose, slightly bent by a boxer's punch.

Regina was a small, pleasant city of sixty thousand people in the forties. The Douglases had moved into a nice, but heavily mortgaged, two-story house at 217 Angus Crescent, a quiet, tree-lined street in the enclave known as the Crescents just across Albert Street and Wascana Lake from the legislature. Tommy would stroll through the area, stopping on his way to work in the morning to chat with neighbours and children on their way to nearby Davin School, where

Shirley and Joan went. In late afternoon, he'd come home, so worn out he could hardly speak on some days. Irma would have supper ready, and she'd take the phone off the hook. "Mom built him not only a castle, but almost a fortress," Joan remembered. "Nothing was allowed to disturb him at home." After eating, he would invariably have a nap, then often go back to his office for another few hours.

Saturday mornings were just like others at the premier's office, but the afternoons were dedicated to party business. Carlyle King, the University of Saskatchewan English professor who was president of the party, would regularly come down for a chat with Tommy, and the two, both pipe smokers, would "blow smoke at each other," as King recalled it. The Douglases occasionally went out to eat on Saturday nights – their favourite spot was the W.K. Chop Suey House on South Railway Avenue. On Sunday, Tommy instructed a Sunday School class at Regina's First Baptist Church and visited sick people in hospital and in nice weather would occasionally bang a ball around the golf course. The premier continued to be a voracious reader – he was fond of Agatha Christie and other mystery writers – but on Sunday afternoons in summer and fall liked nothing better than taking in a Saskatchewan Roughriders game with Irma and the girls.

They rarely entertained. As Tom McLeod put it: Tommy "had a million friends, but not very many really close."

More for recreation than business, he went partners with Clarence Fines in a mink farm that lost money, and later invested in a drive-in movie, Regina's first. Opposition wags dubbed it "the premier's passion pit," and he had to get out after there was a scandal involving another partner.

Soon after his election, Tommy set his sights on a trip overseas to visit Saskatchewan troops. His first attempt, in November 1944, got him no farther than Ottawa, where he took sick and landed in hospital. The hospital stay cost a thousand dollars, which he had to borrow.

He tried again the following March, sailing on a troop ship through the submarine-infested North Atlantic, which brought back vivid memories of crossing the same dangerous waters as a child returning to Scotland. He wandered around Europe on his own for a couple of months, visiting Canadian troops wherever he could find them. At one hospital, at a loss for words, he blurted out: "Well, fellows, I can certainly understand why you like this hospital. All the prettiest girls in Canada must have been shipped over here to look after you." That went over well, but a newspaper report of his visit earned him the cold shoulder from women back home. Irma never let him forget that foot-in-the-mouth.

The highlight of his trip came when he managed to finagle a sneak visit to the South Saskatchewan Regiment deep in Germany, where the war was dragging on. On the way back, though, his jeep was in an accident and Tommy was thrown from it, hurting his knee again. Then, on his own, his knee aching, his clothes torn and dirty, he had to walk for miles. From that point on, his knee would continue to bother him periodically, often flaring up in the fall when the weather would turn cool and damp, and would require periods in bed or even in hospital.

Apparently Europe just wasn't good for Tommy's health. Travelling in Italy in 1959, he contracted Bell's palsy, a condition that temporarily paralyzed the right side of his face. Although he looked terrible and he spoke with difficulty, he pressed on with a major speech he had scheduled, and, as usual, turned it into a joke: "This affliction may be the most effective means yet devised for keeping politicians silent. When I return to Canada, I intend to bite several politicians I know in the hope of infecting them."

One politician he really would have liked to bite was Walter Tucker.

∞

The CCF lost ground in the 1948 election, dropping from forty-seven seats to thirty-one, while the Liberals, under their new leader, a former MP, improved from five to nineteen. Tommy believed the setback was the result of too much change, too fast. "Only a small minority might have their toes stepped on," he commented, "but they tend to remember."

The Liberals were also helped by pooling their forces with Conservatives in many ridings, and by a vehement red-baiting campaign. "Tucker or Tyranny" was their slogan, and their leader charged that Tommy followed marching orders from Moscow.

"Nothing can be quite so resentful as a man who has ridden on your back for fifty years and then you make him get off and walk," Tommy quipped about the business community's reaction to his government's reforms.

But even he was taken aback by the vehemence of the attack against the CCF. "I never thought politics could get so dirty. They threw everything they had into it…. We were communists, we were atheists, we were anti-religious, this was the beginning of the Soviet Union being set up in Canada."

Tommy fought back with sweet reason. "There's no lie too preposterous for them to spread, and no tactics too despicable for them to adopt," he told a radio audience. "Don't let them deceive you again. If they fool you once, shame on them. If they fool you twice…shame on you."

Despite the setback, Tommy had an easy time personally with Tucker, a large, heavyset man who was no match for the premier's lightning wit. During a debate at a Crystal Lake picnic in the summer of 1947, before a boisterous crowd of three thousand, Tucker mentioned a Liberal achievement accomplished, he said, when the premier was "just a little fellow."

"I am still a little fellow," Tommy shot back. "Tucker is big enough to swallow me, but if he did he would be the strangest man in the world because he would have more brains in his stomach than he has in his head."

Tucker continued to be a thorn in Tommy's side, suing him for slander at one point (Tommy won, but it put him in debt), and raising allegations of kickbacks against Fines in 1953. That produced the government's one real scandal, although Fines was cleared by an inquiry and the whole case dismissed for lack of evidence. When Tucker continued to press the issue in the legislature, Tommy lost his temper and, in a blistering speech that lasted almost three hours, tore the charges to shreds and challenged Liberal MLAs who really believed Fines was guilty of anything to stand up. "Come out of the bushes and let's see the colour of your liver!" he mocked them.

Tucker retired from politics soon afterward.

The stain of the scandal stuck to Fines, though, and gossip about him accelerated after he resigned in 1960 and moved to Florida, a wealthy man. Unfortunately for his reputation, he had quietly amassed a small bundle in stocks and other investments, all legitimate, during his years as treasurer.

The CCF had come to power in Saskatchewan in 1944 on a wave of optimism fuelled by the end of the Depression and the imminent end to the war. The province was in bad shape, and Tommy promised to fix it. It's debatable how committed the voters ever were to socialism, no matter the zeal of the party's leaders and stalwarts.

By 1950, with most of its initial campaign promises enacted, the economy on an even keel, and the move to modernize the province well under way, the fires of radical change were burning low. Tommy knew it and many others in the party knew it too. The people of Saskatchewan looked to Tommy Douglas for good government, not the overthrow of the established system.

Ironically, Tommy had become the head of that established system, in Saskatchewan at least. Although the Saskatchewan Liberals continued to compare him to Lenin, Stalin, and Hitler, most people recognized Tommy as a first-rate leader, "a dreamer and a humanitarian, incorruptible, genuine and intellectually honest," as a visiting Vancouver journalist described him in 1960.

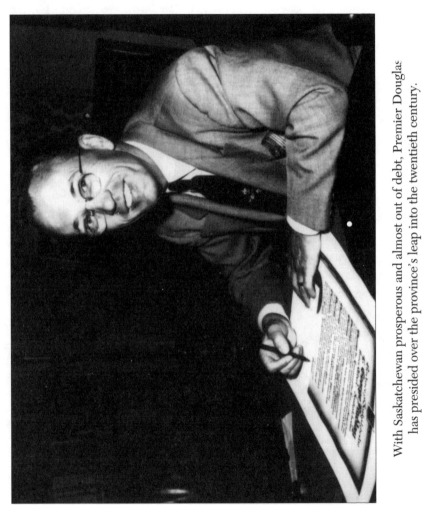

With Saskatchewan prosperous and almost out of debt, Premier Douglas has presided over the province's leap into the twentieth century.

10

The Battle Over Medicare

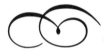

A nother yarn Tommy liked to spin: soon after the 1944 election, he pays a visit to the mental hospital at Weyburn, where he meets a patient walking alone on the grounds.

"How are you sir, and what is your name?"

"Oh, fine," the patient said. "My name is Bob. Who are you?"

"Oh, I'm Tommy Douglas. You know, the premier of Saskatchewan."

The patient gives him a suspicious glance, then replies: "That's all right, you'll get over it. I thought I was Napoleon when I came here."

Over the years that followed, and especially during the doctors' strike of 1961, Tommy may well have thought he was crazy when he considered the challenges of bringing free medical care to every resident of Saskatchewan. But it was the one thing he most wanted to accomplish.

Doing it proved to be his greatest fight, and his greatest achievement, leading eventually to the adoption of a publicly funded universal health care insurance plan nationally.

The struggle, which erupted into national headlines in 1961 with a bitter strike by doctors, had actually been going on since the CCF was first elected in 1944. In fact, the idea for some sort of medicare scheme had been around in Saskatchewan since the twenties, when many towns had a salaried doctor, and had been mentioned in the CCF's 1933 Regina Manifesto.

Tommy had never forgotten his own medical experiences as a boy, when his leg was saved only through the charity of a doctor, and the plight of his parishioners in Weyburn during the Depression, too broke to seek the care of a doctor, was also still fresh in his mind. As he told the legislature, "I made a pledge that if I ever have anything to do with it, people would be able to get health services just as they are able to get educational services, as an inalienable right of being a citizen."

When he handed out cabinet posts, he took the minister of health's job for himself, and immediately set out to improve the state of health care in the province. One of his first steps was to appoint a commission to study the province's needs, and by the fall of 1944 there was a report on Tommy's desk calling for adoption of a system under which every citizen would have the right to free medical care. Tommy sensed that the public was in favour of such a plan – all that remained was the money to finance it. Finding the financial resources would take over fifteen years.

In the meantime, Tommy set in motion a variety of smaller reforms: free medical care for some thirty thousand single mothers, widows, and old people; free treatment for cancer and psychiatric problems; an air ambulance service, the first in the country. The government even gave aid for the gradual installation of running water in towns and villages, marking the beginning of the end for the unhygienic privy. A medical school was opened at the University of Saskatchewan, and improvements were made to the treatment of mental patients. Health districts were established, and the government set in motion a hospital building program that doubled the number of hospital beds in the province within a decade, taking Saskatchewan from last in the country, on a per capita basis, to first.

By the start of 1947, Tommy had launched a provincewide program of free hospital care – the first patient to enroll under the program, shortly after midnight on January 1, was a woman about to deliver a baby. The program cost $7.5 million, or 15 per cent of the provincial budget, that first year, and it had risen to $29 million, or 20 per cent of the budget, by 1955. To help defray the cost, there was a premium of five dollars per person or ten dollars per family, and a limited

sales tax was enacted. Tommy reassured hospital officials worried about government interference: "We have
enough to look after without worrying about whether
or not the bedpans in Tisdale are clean."

Despite all these advances, the dream of a full
health insurance plan remained elusive – with
Saskatchewan still deeply in debt, it was just too expen-
sive. But, starting in 1958, after years of paying lip service to the idea, the federal government, with
Diefenbaker prime minister, began to chip in half of
the Saskatchewan hospital plan. The following April,
Tommy announced his decision to forge ahead with full
medicare.

"If we can do this," he boasted, "then I would like
to hazard the prophecy that before 1970 almost every
other province in Canada will have followed our lead."

He promised a committee would be set up to
determine the best shape for the plan, and that nothing
would be done without the approval of the province's
doctors. It was a promise that became impossible to
fulfill.

Saskatchewan's doctors and their organization, the
College of Physicians and Surgeons, had been opposed
to a public health plan from day one, unless it was a
fee-for-service plan and they had control of it. Many in
the CCF wanted a program under which doctors would
go on salary, but Tommy conceded on this point and
agreed to fee-for-service. But control was something
the government couldn't give up.

Tommy was convinced that doctors would come
around under the pressure of public opinion. He seriously underestimated them.

The doctors dragged their heels in negotiations, and later, their members on the committee Tommy set up to study the issue played dog in the manger.

Tommy called their bluff by making medicare the key issue in the June 1960 election. "The people of this province will decide whether or not we want a medical care program," he told the doctors. In retaliation, the doctors raised a war chest of $100,000, much of it donated by the American Medical Association, and launched a massive advertising campaign, claiming the CCF planned to put doctors on salary, that doctors would leave the province en masse, and that the government would bring in "the garbage of Europe" to fill their shoes. They claimed doctor-patient confidentiality would disappear, that patients with hard-to-diagnose problems would be shipped off to insane asylums by bungling bureaucrats.

Saskatchewan voters don't scare easily, and they returned the CCF with a solid majority. It was "a little short of a political miracle," Tommy said.

Despite the election results, the doctors continued to stall on the advisory committee, and Tommy was reluctant to move without its approval. Walter Erb, who had been appointed health minister after the 1956 election, was the wrong man for the job and was doing more harm than good in his shuttling back and forth between the government and the doctors. A year passed without serious developments.

In August 1961, the equation changed drastically when Tommy won the leadership of the newly established New Democratic Party and his resignation as premier was imminent. He called a special session of the legislature to enact medicare. At the same time, the doctors dug in their heels, voting overwhelmingly on October 13 to defy the law.

On. November 1, Tommy stepped down as premier, and his long-time education minister, Woodrow Lloyd, was selected to replace him. Lloyd set April 1, 1962, as the startup date for medicare and re-opened talks with the doctors, later pushing the deadline back to July 1. When that day came, the doctors, who were emboldened by the government's frequent delays, went on strike, aided by dozens of Liberal-supported Keep Our Doctors committees that sprang up a across the province.

Replacement doctors were brought in, flown in by the planeload, many of them from Britain, and the strike, bitter as it was, lost steam. By the end of the month, an agreement had been reached and the doctors were back at work. Medicare was a reality at long last, and quickly became accepted by almost all. In 1967, the federal government would enact a funding plan that brought medicare to all the provinces. It was an idea whose time had clearly come – Saskatchewan was just five years ahead of the country.

But it was in this overheated environment of crisis that Tommy Douglas suffered his first defeat at the polls since his first run for office in 1934. Diefenbaker called a federal election for June 1962 and Tommy, as new leader of the NDP, ran in Regina, where he was beaten.

And, in April 1964, Lloyd and his government were thrown out by Ross Thatcher, a one-time CCF member of Parliament who had become leader of the Saskatchewan Liberals. Some people blamed the fight over medicare, others Tommy's departure, others the simple fact that the government was twenty years old, and the people felt it was time for a change.

Tommy, as always, looked on the bright side. He recalled how the early Christians had their greatest success after they began to be persecuted and many of them "were scattered abroad teaching the Gospel," as the New Testament put it.

"In other words," Tommy said, "what looked like a terrible tragedy scattered them out over the world of that day. Instead of sitting around and holding hands with each other and saying what a wonderful group they were, they were forced to go out and talk to other people."

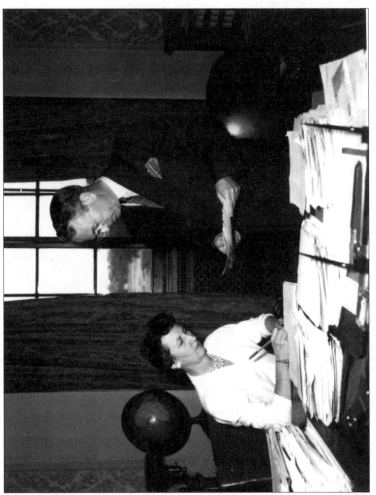

Douglas works with his secretary, Eleanor McKinnon, in 1961, the same year Saskatchewan enacts medicare and he resigns as premier to become leader of the NDP.

11

A New Challenge, and Putting Down the Sword

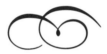

A sweltering night in August, 1961, Ottawa, a crowded coliseum. Tommy Douglas stands at the podium, his arms raised, his trademark smile plastered across his face, listening to thunderous applause.

This founding convention of the New Democratic Party (NDP) is a political convention like none the Co-operative Commonwealth Federation (CCF) ever held. Those were sober, staid gatherings devoted to resolutions and debate. At this one, music, buttons, balloons, and banners help create a flavour of show-biz hoopla. Delegates sing a newly written song, "A Douglas for Me." It's the biggest political convention ever staged in Canada, with over two thousand delegates shouting Tommy's name, and it's the first bilingual one.

Tommy looks into the television cameras and tells Canadians what this new party he's just been chosen to lead can offer them. There's no mention of an end to capitalism, but he calls for free health care and education, public pensions, a new commitment to world peace. The next election, he vows, will be fought under the banner of "free enterprise versus socialism."

Come join us, he invites Canadians. "We haven't plumbed the depths and found all the answers. We want new ideas. We want eventually to establish a people's government."

And as the music rises again, he urges his audience to join him in a slightly modified version of one of his favourite quotes from the British poet, William Blake:

> I shall not cease from mental strife,
> Nor shall my sword rest in my hand,
> Till we have built Jerusalem,
> In this green and pleasant land.

Flash forward ten months. Regina, a mild night in June, a light rain falling. Tommy and Irma have spent some of the worst hours of their lives, at the Hotel Saskatchewan, watching the election results roll in: only nineteen New Democrats elected to Parliament across the nation – not a single one from Saskatchewan – as the Diefenbaker Tories sweep the West and the Liberals own the East. The final blow: Tommy himself going down to a humiliating defeat in Regina, trounced by almost a ten-thousand-vote margin.

The former five-time premier of Saskatchewan looks small, almost frail, as he and his wife walk hand in hand through the rain to their green Pontiac. The streets are almost deserted as they drive to the television station on the eastern edge of the city, where Tommy, quoting an old Scottish ballad with calm dignity, will tell the province and nation, "I'll lay me down and bleed a while, and then I'll rise and fight again."

Then it's home to Angus Crescent, tea and raisin toast, and bed.

∞

The CCF was, if anything, a victim of its own success. Its radical agenda made sense to a lot of people with the war in the daily headlines and the Depression fresh in memory. Twenty years later, an affluent, peaceful society saw little need to change from the two established parties, parties that had adopted some CCF ideas, and, except in Saskatchewan, the CCF became increasingly marginalized.

Even before the shock of the 1958 federal election, which reduced the caucus to eight seats and left even Coldwell and Knowles without jobs, there had been talk of a new alliance of the CCF with organized labour. That jolt only intensified the organizing for such a union, led by Knowles and David Lewis, the party national president. Tommy Douglas was ambivalent. He knew the CCF must widen its appeal nationally but was reluctant to give up on what had been achieved in Saskatchewan. Still, the kinship between farmers and unionists seemed self-evident to him: "The farmer...needs allies," he told a farmers' group. "And where can he find them? Only among the men and women who sell the products of their labour just as you sell the products of your labour." But the bonds between farm and union that had helped bring the CCF together almost thirty years earlier had frayed. The new party being discussed back East had the potential to restore those bonds, and, by edging the party more toward the centre, appeal to liberal-minded Canadians who weren't interested in socialism.

Tommy was less ambivalent about the leadership of the new party – he didn't want it. In Saskatchewan, he was popular, he had real power, and there was potential to do much more good work. On the national scene, well, as a CCF member of Parliament, he had been "almost overcome with the frustration and futility of being a voice crying in the wilderness," he wrote to a friend.

Despite his denials, Tommy had long been regarded as Coldwell's natural heir. Lewis and Knowles wanted him, as did many other leaders within the CCF and the unions. Petitions from across the country poured into Tommy's office, pleading with him to take the job, and even Irma told her husband he had "a real responsibility" to the national movement.

Tommy wavered. "Frankly, I'm not keen about entering the federal field," he wrote to his cabinet pal John Brockelbank. "My colleagues here have been so pleasant to work with, and the job is so fascinating, I'd like nothing better than staying here in Saskatchewan." What's more, he had "no illusions about our achieving government in Canada in my lifetime. But if I can help lay the foundations for a movement that will ultimately establish economic democracy in Canada, it would be a worthwhile contribution."

What ultimately decided him was that the only other serious candidate was Hazen Argue, a CCF MP from Saskatchewan who Tommy thought would be a poor choice. He was also concerned about the visible drift to the right in Canadian politics. He wanted, he said, to offer voters "a genuine choice between progressive and reactionary policies." He was convinced that, in his own small way, he could bring some of the magic of the Saskatchewan CCF experience to the new party and the nation.

∞

The new phase of Tommy's life got off to a bad start. He'd easily won the leadership of the New Democratic Party over Argue, who a few months later would desert the party for the Liberals, the first of a series of jolts for the new leader. Tommy resigned as premier of Saskatchewan and set off across the country trying to build up some excitement for the NDP. But there was a string of by-election defeats for the new "labour" party in Ontario – union leaders may have supported it, but rank and file workers were not convinced, and their much vaunted vote failed to materialize.

Then came the calamity of June 1962, with the party's poor showing in the federal election and his own bitter defeat.

Tommy's campaign in Regina foreshadowed what was in store for the party. The city's residents had been whipped into a near-hysteria by the doctors' anti-medicare campaign, and voters were angry at Tommy, paradoxically, both for his role in advancing the health care plan and for "deserting" the province.

There were graffiti threats on city walls and calls in the middle of the night to Tommy's house. His campaign manager, Ed Whelan, got frequent calls from a man threatening to "shoot you, you Red bastard!" Tommy's motorcade in the city's west side was booed by angry Keep Our Doctor pickets, some of whom spit, made the Nazi salute or threw stones at his car. A few homeowners placed symbolic coffins on their front lawns. Tommy had never seen anything like it.

The defeat that followed, according to daughter Shirley, hurt him like nothing else ever had; it "was the most terrible thing that ever happened."

He had only a short time to lick his wounds after the Regina debacle, though. Erhart Regier, a New Democrat MP in British Columbia and Douglas loyalist, resigned his seat in Burnaby-Coquitlam, forcing a by-election, which Tommy won handily. He returned to the same sixth-floor office in Parliament's Centre Block where he'd begun his political career almost thirty years earlier.

Eleanor McKinnon, his faithful secretary, followed him and Irma to Ottawa, but the girls were out on their own. Shirley was in England, where she'd studied at the Royal Academy of Dramatic Arts and stayed on, pursuing an acting career – her first movie role was in the controversial *Lolita*. She had married, and the Douglases now had their first grandson, another Thomas, known as Tad. Joan, who later would marry and move to Israel, was in her fourth year of nursing at the University of Saskatchewan.

∞

At the end of his seventeen years in Saskatchewan, Tommy was, if anything, more radical than ever, and to those who thought he'd mellowed he said "absolute nonsense." He was eager to apply the lessons of Saskatchewan to the whole country. "In 1944, I thought these things could be done," he said, "and today I know they *can* be done." He rattled off a list of his accomplishments. "All these things are now accepted as part of our way of life in this province. We've become convinced that these things, which were once thought to be radical, aren't radical at all; they're just plain common sense applied to the economic and social problems of our times."

His failure to achieve any of these successes on the national scene was a source of continual frustration and bitter disappointment to Tommy and his supporters over the next decade. Through a succession of elections, the New Democrats under his leadership were never able to elect more than two dozen MPs or to break out of their marginalized position in Parliament, though they did hold the balance of power in two minority governments – a chip Tommy perhaps played badly when they contributed to the defeat of Diefenbaker and the resurgence of the Liberals in 1963. Between supporting Tories or Liberals, "it is like having to choose between being hanged or shot," he said, dubbing Diefenbaker and Lester Pearson "Tweedledum and Tweedledee."

After his 1962 rebuff in Regina, some of Tommy's spark seemed to desert him, but he remained one of the most effective campaigners in Canada and always drew huge crowds. And, despite the party's position on the sidelines, Tommy now had become truly a national figure. The NDP functioned as the conscience of Parliament in the Diefenbaker and Pearson years, just as the CCF had for King and St. Laurent, often nudging the government leftward. While Tommy was leader of the NDP, Pearson's Liberals brought in medicare, the Canada Pension Plan, and labour reforms similar to those adopted in Saskatchewan twenty years earlier.

In a 1970 speech, he asked rhetorically if his life had been wasted. After all, the NDP hadn't even come close to power federally. Tommy shook his head. "I look back and think that a boy from a poor home on the wrong side of the tracks in Winnipeg was given the privilege of being part of a movement that has changed Canada. In my lifetime, I have seen it change Canada."

Indeed, toward the end of Tommy's career, political columnist Charles Lynch wrote that "as much as any man, it was Douglas who turned Canada into the most highly socialized country in the Western world, without anybody really noticing what was happening."

Hardly a waste.

The NDP was also a constant thorn in the government's left side on questions of nationalism, economic development, NATO, and other international issues. It was Tommy's idea to have a commission to study bilingualism and multiculturalism, and he played a key role in finding compromise in the bitter debate over a new Canadian flag. Tommy and most of his caucus stood alone in protesting Prime Minister Pierre Trudeau's use of the War Measures Act during the 1970 Quebec crisis. The sight of tanks rolling in Ottawa immediately reminded him of the police riots in Winnipeg and Estevan he'd witnessed, and of Nazis goose-stepping in Germany. It sent shivers down his back.

Tommy deplored the kidnappings and supported legitimate government actions to deal with the situation. But, he told the House, to cries of "Shame!" from Liberals and Tories, the government "is using a sledgehammer to crack a peanut." The NDP, he said, was "not prepared to use the preservation of law and order as a smokescreen to destroy the liberties and the freedoms of the people of Canada."

Tommy's courageous stand on the crisis caused sharp divisions within the party and brought him much abuse. But a documentary film by Donald Brittain later referred to this as "perhaps his finest hour, certainly his loneliest."

During the turbulent sixties, when Tommy was an outspoken critic of U.S. policies in Vietnam and Canada's sympathetic policies, he became popular with young protesters. Not all, though. At one antiwar rally in front of Parliament, he personally intervened when two groups of demonstrators got into a shouting and shoving match. One of the hotheads was swinging a two-by-four at a young woman when the one-time lightweight champion of Manitoba, on hand to deliver a speech, wrestled it from his hands.

Tommy's appeal to the young radical crowd increased when Shirley, working in films in California and remarried to the Hollywood star Donald

Sutherland, was arrested and charged with storing bombs in her home on behalf of the militant Black Panther Party, although no bombs were actually found. Shirley had helped raise funds for the Panthers' free breakfast program for poor children in the Los Angeles slums. Tommy told the Ottawa press he was sure she was innocent and that he was "proud of the fact that my daughter believes, as I do, that hungry children should be fed, whether they are Black Panthers or white Republicans."

After flying to L.A. to be with Shirley, Tommy wrote to a friend that he'd always "thought American society was sick. After being there, I feel that it is nigh unto death." As for Shirley, the charges were thrown out by a judge, but U.S. immigration officials attempted to deport her. She eventually returned to Canada and was blackballed from further work in the U.S., although her son, Kiefer, followed his dad to Hollywood stardom.

∞

In 1968, the Liberals chose Pierre Trudeau, a popular young former New Democrat with a dashing image, as their leader. Within the NDP, there began to be a sentiment for a younger leader as well, even though the party's popularity was rising. When word got to Tommy, he was disappointed but agreed to step aside at the next convention. Before that could happen, though, Trudeau called an election for June. Tommy stole the show in a televised three-way debate with Trudeau and Tory leader Robert Stanfield, but Trudeaumania swept the nation, except in Saskatchewan, where the NDP staged a comeback. Even Tommy was upended, losing his previously comfortable Burnaby seat by a mere 138 votes. He was sixty-three, still vigorous, but it looked like the end of his career. David Lewis, who won a seat in Toronto and had clear ambitions to succeed Tommy, took over as House leader.

There was the usual talk of a sitting MP making way for the fallen leader to run in a by-election, as had happened in 1962. Tommy said no. But fate wasn't through with him yet. Barely a month after the election, Colin Cameron, a veteran Vancouver Island socialist MP, died. Tommy was immediately drafted to run in Nanaimo-Cowichan-The Islands. The Liberals pulled out the stops to beat him, but by the following February, after a rough campaign, he was back in Ottawa, in his old leader's seat.

For the next two years, Tommy stayed on as the party's leader, a pretty vigorous lame-duck – in 1970, his last full year as leader, he travelled 140,000 kilometres, criss-crossing the country. Hans Brown, his assistant at the time, said that Tommy "worked at a ferocious pace and he liked to be sure that everybody else was working ferociously too." He was ready to step aside, but party members, including some people who a year earlier had urged him to resign, pressed him to stay longer. Ironically, this was a period of tremendous victories for the party in the West: NDP governments were elected in Manitoba, under Ed Schreyer, in 1969; Saskatchewan, under Allan Blakeney, a former protégé of Tommy's, in 1971; and British Columbia, under David Barrett, in 1972.

Eventually, the party selected David Lewis as leader and Tommy stepped down after twenty-seven straight years of party leadership. He had run in fourteen elections (six provincially, eight federally), winning eleven. But he was far from through with politics, and would win two more elections, in 1972 and '74, before finally retiring.

Though no longer the leader, Tommy barely slowed down. He always paid close attention to his riding, going home every other week. The people of Vancouver Island rewarded him with 71 per cent of the vote in 1972. He'd already taken on the job as NDP energy critic, and through the seventies, the era of the OPEC oil embargo and skyrocketing oil prices, he was a constant pain in the Trudeau government's backside on energy issues. The National Energy Policy championed by Trudeau, and the creation of a national oil company, Petro-Canada, were very much products of ideas put forward first by Tommy. And it was while he was making an impassioned speech against the Liberals' Syncrude policies in 1975 that Tommy was taken ill, collapsed with a bleeding ulcer, and had to be rushed from the House on a stretcher.

∞

One last hurrah. The NDP's 1983 convention, Regina. It's the fiftieth anniversary of the Regina Manifesto. An ailing, cancer-stricken Tommy Douglas is wheeled into the hall on a golf cart pulling a cake with fifty candles. Tommy is helped onto the stage, his hands trembling. But when they grip the podium, he steadies, and when he begins to speak, his voice is as strong as ever. He gives his audience a brief history lesson, reminding them of Woodsworth, Coldwell, Williams, and of the party's many achievements. But that isn't enough, he tells them. He reminds his listeners that unemployment and poverty still plague Canada, that the gap between rich and poor has widened, that discrimination and hatred still stain the land.

"We're not just interested in getting votes," he admonishes the New Democrats. "We are seeking to get people who are willing to dedicate their lives to building a different kind of society...a society founded on the principles of concern for human well-being and human welfare.

"If I could press a button tonight and bring a million people into this party, and knew that those people were coming in for some ulterior motive but they didn't understand the kind of society we're trying to build, I wouldn't press the button because we don't want those kind of people."

The applause begins before he's barely finished, several thousand people on their feet. It continues for half an hour.

∞

Tommy resigned from Parliament in 1979, at seventy-four. He was still vigorous, and he remained active. He took on the job of chairman of the Douglas-Coldwell Foundation, formed in 1971 as a left-wing think tank, and he led a delegation to China in 1979. As a speaker, he was just as much in demand as ever, and he often wrote articles for magazines, though he resisted numerous entreaties to put his memoirs onto paper. He and Irma spent more time at their cottage in the Gatineau Hills, near Ottawa, often in the company of their grandchildren. Tommy liked to chop wood and take the occasional swim – he invariably could go faster and farther than the kids. In winter, he and Irma liked brief holidays in Jamaica where, in 1972, he had made headlines by socking a man who tried to hold them up.

The discovery, in 1981, that he had an inoperable cancer, slowed him down somewhat, but he remained active. He took a walk every day, and when he was in Ottawa, he always had a fried egg sandwich on brown toast and a pot of tea for lunch at the Colonnade Restaurant on Metcalfe Street.

One hot summer afternoon in 1984, while out for his walk, he stepped carelessly into the path of a city bus, which sent him flying. He was in hospital for weeks but, after a period of touch and go, was able to joke: "If you think I'm in bad shape, you should see the bus."

Back on his feet, he was able to make a last visit to Regina, on December 5, 1985, with his granddaughter Rachel, to receive the Saskatchewan Award of Merit. He'd already been granted numerous honourary degrees and was a Companion of the Order of Canada, and was, he joked, finally "becoming respectable." The Regina trip was his final public appearance, but he paid one last visit to Parliament Hill a few weeks later, for a haircut at the MPs' barbershop where he'd been a regular for over twenty years. Shirley, who drove him, said the outing took all Tommy's strength but he was pleased with the fuss the barbers and Parliament staff made over him. A few weeks later, on February 24, 1986, he died, at last putting down the sword placed in his hands so many years before.

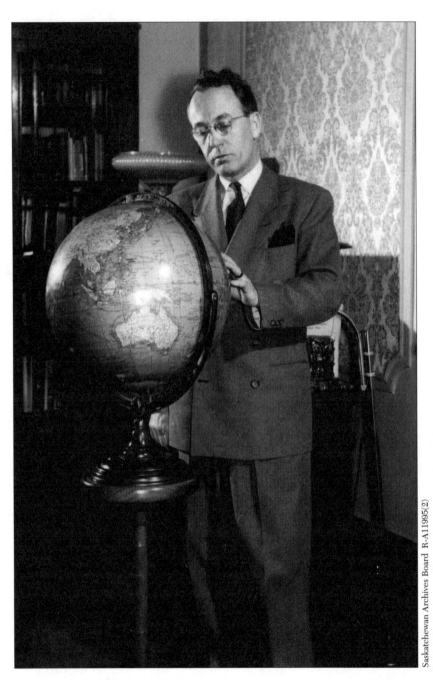

"Our task is to build a new society which has learned to put 'first things first' and to measure progress not in material terms alone."
– Tommy Douglas

Epilogue

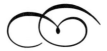

F inally, how to judge Tommy? There've been many accolades, many attempts to pin him to a board like a butterfly and explain him. Here are just a few:

Frank Scott, the Montreal poet and lawyer who had been part of the CCF's early-day brain trust, looked back and compared Tommy to Woodsworth and Coldwell. They "were quite different in their characters and their capabilities," Scott said. "Woodsworth was the philosophical and spiritual leader of the movement, an inspiring figure, but...not the mover of masses. Coldwell also was a somewhat retiring person on the public platform...not terribly effective – fundamentally a parliamentarian, happiest in the House of Commons....

"But Tommy was IT. Tommy related the whole thing to people, to every type of person. He knew how to speak to them, to get their interest, and use his enormous gift of wit and humour to the greatest advantage. He was never very terrifying in his ideas even when putting forth bold CCF policy and he was able to put it into words that made it seem perfectly sensible and reasonable to ordinary people. And he was, therefore, the best."

Bill Davies, a colleague of Tommy's in the Saskatchewan cabinet, summed him up this way: "There are so many things that are deemed worthwhile and talked about that are never done. Tommy Douglas talked about things and did them."

Let's give the last words to a professional word-smith, *Vancouver Sun* columnist Jack Scott, writing in 1960: "Forget the politics. Here's a man who wanted to do something for the improvement of the human race. He chose the method that seemed best to him, quarrel with it if you will. He was motivated by an ideal. To call him a politician, as you'd call Bennett or Diefenbaker politicians, is to insult him."

Tommy was, Scott wrote with succinctness and eloquence the preacher-turned-politician himself would have appreciated, "a good deed in a naughty world...."

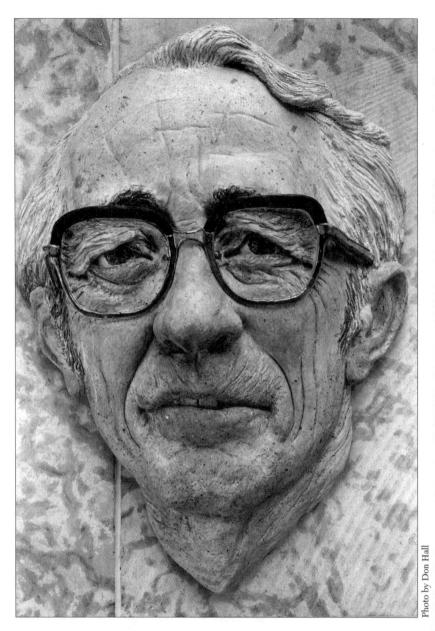

This ceramic head of Tommy Douglas by sculptor Joe Fafard graces the
lobby of the T.C. Douglas Building in Regina, which houses the
Ministry of Health and the Saskatchewan Arts Board.

Chronology of
Tommy Douglas
(1904-1986)

Compiled by Lynne Bowen

DOUGLAS AND HIS TIMES	CANADA AND THE WORLD
	1844 Modern consumer's co-operative movement begins in Rochdale, England.
	1867 British North America Act establishes the Dominion of Canada.
	Canadian Medical Association is created.
	1870 Manitoba becomes a province in the Dominion of Canada.
	1873 Winnipeg, Manitoba, is incorporated as a city.

DOUGLAS AND HIS TIMES	CANADA AND THE WORLD
	1759 Great Iron Works established at Falkirk, Scotland; several generations of the Douglas family will be employed here.
	1880s The Social Gospel urges Canadian Christians to focus on the here rather than the hereafter.
	1881 Formation of the Social Democratic Federation marks the beginning of the Socialist movement in Britain.
	1893 Keir Hardie, a Scot, founds the Independent Labour Party in Britain.
	1898 In Britain, William Gladstone, a former Liberal Prime Minister, dies.
1899-1902 Tom Douglas (Tommy Douglas's father) serves in British Army during the Boer War; when he comes home, he joins the Labour Party; his father, a lifelong Liberal and disciple of Gladstone, throws him out.	**1899-1902** Boer War is fought in South Africa between the British and the Afrikaners; Canada sends troops; the war divides Canadians along French and English lines.
	1901 In Canada, dissatisfaction with the handling of a bumper crop causes Prairie farmers to form the Territorial Grain Growers' Association (TGG).

DOUGLAS AND HIS TIMES	CANADA AND THE WORLD
1904 Thomas Clement Douglas is born on October 20 in Falkirk, Scotland; his grandfather comes "to see the boy" and is reconciled with the boy's father; the entire family eventually joins the Labour Party.	**1904** James Shaver Woodsworth (future leader of the Co-operative Commonwealth Federation) works with immigrant slum dwellers in Winnipeg's All People's Mission and advocates the Social Gospel.
	1905 Alberta and Saskatchewan become provinces of Canada.
	1906 TGG divides into the Saskatchewan Grain Growers' Association (SGG) and the Alberta Farmers' Association. The British Labour Party wins twenty-nine seats.
1908 Stanley Knowles (future friend and colleague of Tommy Douglas) is born in Los Angeles, California.	**1908** Retired British General Robert Baden-Powell founds the Boy Scouts.
1910 Tom Douglas, Sr. emigrates to Canada ahead of his wife and children and ends up in Winnipeg, Manitoba. Weakened by pneumonia, Tommy Douglas injures his right knee in a fall; the onset of osteomyelitis makes several operations necessary.	

DOUGLAS AND HIS TIMES

1911
In early spring, Tommy Douglas, his sister Annie, and his pregnant mother, Anne, leave Glasgow for Canada; a seventeen-day sea voyage and a five-day train ride bring them to Winnipeg, where his father has rented a house in the North End; Douglas's second sister, Isobel, is born.

1912-1914
Douglas is hospitalized often for treatment to his knee; Dr. R.H. Smith saves Douglas's leg with an experimental surgical procedure, one that the Douglas family could not have afforded on their own.

CANADA AND THE WORLD

1911
Canada's Liberal Prime Minister, Sir Wilfrid Laurier, loses the election to Conservative Robert Borden.

In the previous twenty years, the population of western Canada has grown from 250,000 to 2,000,000, due largely to immigration.

In Britain, Ramsay MacDonald becomes chairman of the Labour Party; the Liberal government introduces the National Health Insurance Act.

1914-1918
Douglas family returns to Scotland where Tom Sr. rejoins the British army; the family lives with Anne's family (the Clements) in Glasgow; Tommy Douglas is influenced by his grandfather's interest in co-ops, and by the preachers he listens to in church and the socialists and other soapbox speakers he hears on Glasgow Green.

1914
Britain declares war on Germany; Canada is automatically at war; British expatriates return to join the armed forces.

First compulsory contributory social insurance legislation in Canada, the Workmen's Compensation Act, is passed in Ontario.

The Social Gospel advocates Prohibition, women's suffrage, civil service reform, and co-operatives.

1916
First mothers' allowance legislation in Canada is passed in Manitoba.

1917
At the Battle of Vimy Ridge in April, Canadian soldiers fight as a unit for the first time and achieve victory where the British and French have failed.

Conscription divides Canadians along French/English lines and leads to the formation of the Union government, which offers the vote to female relatives of soldiers.

In the October Revolution in Russia, the Bolshevik (later the Communist) Party seizes power.

DOUGLAS AND HIS TIMES	CANADA AND THE WORLD
	1918
	Armistice ends World War I in November.
	Worldwide influenza epidemic kills almost twenty-two million people in two years.
1919	**1919**
Tommy Douglas, his mother, and two sisters sail for Canada on January 1; Douglas is "the man of the family" until his father can join them.	Treaty of Versailles is signed.
	In the Winnipeg General Strike, 35,000 workers leave their jobs; federal government officials co-operate with the employers; Royal North-West Mounted Police charge a crowd on "Bloody Saturday" (June 21) leaving one dead and twenty-nine injured; federal troops occupy Winnipeg; J.S. Woodsworth is among those arrested.
Douglas family buys a house at 132 McPhail Street, Winnipeg.	
Tommy Douglas and Mark Talnicoff (later Talney, Douglas's future brother-in-law) watch "Bloody Saturday" from the roof of a two-story building.	
	The One Big Union (OBU), a new revolutionary industrial union, receives overwhelming acceptance by mine, transportation, and logging workers mostly in Western Canada.
Having quit school in Scotland, Douglas begins a printer's apprenticeship; in his spare time he joins the Boy Scouts, the Order of DeMolay, and the militia; he studies music, boxing, elocution, and acting; he reads Sir Walter Scott and Robert Burns and political and religious books.	

DOUGLAS AND HIS TIMES

1920
Douglas is the youngest Linotype operator in Canada.

1920-1924
Douglas performs at Burns dinners and concerts; he takes over the leading role in a play and receives a standing ovation; he is a lay preacher at Stonewall, Manitoba.

1921
Douglas begins boxing at a gym operated by the OBU.

CANADA AND THE WORLD

1920
Ontario and Prairie farmers unite with dissident Liberals led by Thomas Crerar to form the Progressive Party.

Canada joins the newly formed League of Nations.

Unemployment insurance is introduced in Great Britain and Austria.

1921
In the first federal election in which women have the vote, Agnes Macphail is the only woman elected; the Progressive Party wins sixty-five seats and permanently breaks the two-party pattern of federal politics; William Lyon Mackenzie King becomes the Liberal prime minister.

Communist Party of Canada is founded in Guelph, Ontario.

Tommy Douglas

DOUGLAS AND HIS TIMES	CANADA AND THE WORLD

1922

Douglas wins the amateur lightweight boxing championship of Manitoba.

1922

In Britain, unemployed Glasgow workers undertake a hunger march on London.

In Italy, Mussolini marches on Rome and later forms a fascist government.

Union of Soviet Socialist Republics (U.S.S.R.) is formed from the Russian empire.

1924

Douglas enrolls at Brandon College, where the Social Gospel thrives, to finish high school and study theology; he supports himself with public speaking, waiting on tables, and preaching; he is assigned to the Presbyterian Church in Carberry, Manitoba, where Irma Dempsey (his future wife) comes to hear him preach.

1924

The Labour Party under Ramsay MacDonald forms the first left-wing government in Britain.

The Communist Party of Canada abandons secrecy and changes its name to the Workers' Party.

The Saskatchewan Wheat Pool begins operations and adds impetus to the province's growing co-op movement.

DOUGLAS AND HIS TIMES	CANADA AND THE WORLD

1925

Douglas meets Stanley Knowles and they become academic rivals and lifelong friends.

1925

In the United States (U.S.) the Scopes (or Monkey) Trial in Tennessee pits fundamentalists against scientists over the origin of humankind; several professors at Brandon College are cleared of heresy charges for being on the side of science.

The United Church is formed in Canada; it is partly a product of the Social Gospel, by now in decline.

Unemployment Insurance Act enacted in Britain.

1926

Tommy Douglas is assigned as a lay preacher to Baptist churches in Shoal Lake and Strathclair.

1926

Combining the radical Farmers' Union of Canada and the SGG, the United Farmers of Canada (Saskatchewan Section) or the UFC (SS) is established.

James Garfield (Jimmy) Gardiner first elected Premier of Saskatchewan.

In Britain there is a general strike.

1927

Old Age Pension legislation is passed in Canada partly due to the efforts of J.S. Woodsworth.

Socialists riot in Vienna; a general strike follows the acquittal of Nazis for a political murder.

DOUGLAS AND HIS TIMES

1928

Irma Dempsey finishes high school and comes to study music at Brandon College, where Douglas is student body president.

1930

Douglas graduates from college and is ordained; he marries Irma Dempsey and they are sent to the Calvary Baptist Church in Weyburn, Saskatchewan; he studies by correspondence toward a master's degree in sociology.

1931

Douglas takes charge of eleven delinquents; businessmen label him a "Red" when he calls for increased relief rates.

In the summer Douglas goes to the University of Chicago for graduate work; he and other students visit a hobo jungle; he attends a meeting of the U.S. Socialist Party and becomes disillusioned by political purists and theorists.

Douglas visits Estevan and Bienfait during the coal miners' strike; he preaches against the shocking living conditions; mine owners complain to Douglas's church deacons.

CANADA AND THE WORLD

1928

Norman Thomas, leader of the Socialist Party in the U.S., is defeated in the first of his six runs for the presidency of the U.S.

1929

U.S. Stock Exchange collapses on October 28, and the ten-year-long Great Depression begins.

1930

In Canada, the federal government finally transfers jurisdiction of Crown lands in Saskatchewan and Alberta to the two provinces.

1931

Coal miners in Bienfait, Saskatchewan, strike on September 8; the press and the government focus on the presence of communists; only the UFC (SS) is sympathetic; a demonstration in nearby Estevan on September 29 is crushed by the Royal Canadian Mounted Police; three miners are killed and twenty-three are injured.

Drought, crop failures, and plummeting wheat prices cause the provincial income to drop by 90 per cent; 66 per cent of the rural population is on relief.

DOUGLAS AND HIS TIMES	CANADA AND THE WORLD
1932	**1932**
At the urging of J.S. Woodsworth, M.J. Coldwell meets Douglas in Weyburn; Douglas becomes president of the new Weyburn branch of Coldwell's Independent Labour Party (ILP).	First U.S. unemployment insurance law is enacted in Wisconsin.
	Franklin Roosevelt elected President of the U.S.; he is re-elected three times.
In July, UFC (SS) and the ILP form the Farmer-Labour Party with M.J. Coldwell as leader; Douglas is elected to the party's council in absentia.	Nazis win a majority in the German Reichstag elections.
1933	**1933**
Co-operative Commonwealth Federation (CCF) is founded under the leadership of J.S. Woodsworth; the convention issues the Regina Manifesto, which contains many radical ideas that are later accepted as part of Canadian life; the manifesto, which Douglas calls "the finest thing I have ever seen," vows to eradicate capitalism.	The gross national product of Canada has declined by 42 per cent since the beginning to the Great Depression; 30 per cent of the work force is unemployed.
	CCF wins six seats in British Columbia (B.C.).
Douglas flirts briefly with "eugenics," a theory for improvement of the race that will lose favour when embraced by the Nazis.	Price of a bushel of wheat has dropped from $1.60 in 1929 to below 40 cents.
	Adolf Hitler is appointed German Chancellor; he suppresses labour unions and harasses Jews.

DOUGLAS AND HIS TIMES	CANADA AND THE WORLD
1934	**1934**
Shirley Douglas (Douglas's daughter) is born in April.	Dionne quintuplets born in Callendar, Ontario.
In June, an inexperienced Douglas places third in his riding in the Saskatchewan election; at the national CCF convention that summer Douglas agrees to lead the party's youth wing.	
1935	**1935**
Douglas studies in Chicago during the summer.	The On to Ottawa Trek ends in the Regina Riot.
Although the Baptist church tells Douglas to stay out of politics, he runs for the CCF in the federal election; worried that the Social Credit will split their votes, the CCF and the Liberals scheme; Douglas wins the seat by 301 votes with his simple style, attention-getting gimmicks, and sense of drama and humour; the CCF wins eight seats, which quickly reduce to five (Woodsworth, Douglas, Coldwell, Grant MacNeil, and Angus MacInnis).	Social Credit Party of William "Bible Bill" Aberhart wins a landslide victory in Alberta and runs candidates in Saskatchewan in the federal election, which is won by Mackenzie King's Liberals; Jimmy Gardiner begins a twenty-two-year term as the minister of agriculture.
	League for Social Reconstruction publishes *Social Planning for Canada*, which advocates expansion of the welfare state.
Douglas resigns as the minister of Calvary Baptist Church in Weyburn, and the family moves to Ottawa.	Nazis repudiate the Versailles Treaty; Mussolini invades Ethiopia.
	Roosevelt signs the U.S. Social Security Act.

DOUGLAS AND HIS TIMES	**CANADA AND THE WORLD**

1936

Tom Douglas Sr. dies of a burst appendix.

Douglas is a delegate at an international youth conference in Geneva; he sees Nazis marching in German streets and realizes force will be necessary to defeat them; this puts him at odds with Woodsworth, who is a pacifist.

In his maiden speech in the House of Commons, Douglas criticizes the government for its inaction when Italy invades Ethiopia.

1937

Drought in southern Saskatchewan is the worst in its history.

1938

Although the CCF doubles its seats to eleven in the Saskatchewan election, there is discontent with the party leadership.

1936

Spanish Civil War begins.

Mussolini and Hitler proclaim the Rome-Berlin Axis.

1937

Quebec passes the Padlock Act, which can be used to evict communists.

Canadians volunteer for the international brigades to assist the communist-supported republican government during the Spanish Civil War.

Japan begins an aggressive war policy and invades China.

1938

Hitler marches into Austria; Britain appeases Germany at Munich.

DOUGLAS AND HIS TIMES

1939

Seeing his communist associates change their rhetoric after Stalin's pact with Hitler, Douglas condemns them in his article "I Am Disgusted."

Pacifist Woodsworth resigns as CCF head; Coldwell becomes leader and Douglas his unofficial lieutenant; CCF attempts unsuccessfully to limit war profiteering.

Douglas enlists in the South Saskatchewan Regiment, is soon given a commission, and rises to a captain.

1940

In the March federal election, Douglas retains his seat in Weyburn; the CCF elects eight, five of them from Saskatchewan.

Tommy and Irma Douglas adopt a second daughter, Joan.

1941

In October, the army transfers Douglas to the Winnipeg Grenadiers; just before his unit is to leave to reinforce the British garrison at Hong Kong in November, he is turned down because of his old leg injury.

CANADA AND THE WORLD

1939

In June, Stalin signs a non-aggression treaty with Hitler; Canadian communists change their anti-fascist rhetoric.

Spanish Civil War ends; Britain and France recognize the fascist government.

World War II begins in September; Canada declares war.

United Mine Workers of America strike in the U.S.

1940

In Canada, the Liberals win a huge majority in March; the Unemployment Insurance Act passes; the War Measures Act bans the Communist Party of Canada, which re-emerges as the Labor-Progressive Party.

1941

CCF is B.C.'s official opposition.

Japan bombs Pearl Harbour on December 7; U.S., Britain, and Canada declare war on Japan; Japan attacks Hong Kong; of the 1975 Canadians there, 557 are killed or die in prison camps.

DOUGLAS AND HIS TIMES

1942
Douglas gains a national profile when he speaks eloquently in the post-Hong Kong furor in Ottawa.

Douglas wins the leadership of the Saskatchewan CCF.

CCF supports the federal government treatment of Japanese-Canadians; Douglas is mostly silent on the issue.

J.S. Woodsworth dies; Stanley Knowles wins his seat in Parliament.

CANADA AND THE WORLD

1942
Progressive Party members join the Conservative Party to form the Progressive Conservative (PC) Party.

U.S. and Canada forcibly move Japanese citizens inland, away from the west coast of North America.

Canadians suffer heavy losses in the failed raid on Dieppe, which was meant to test Hitler's defenses.

1943
CCF is Ontario's official opposition.

Germany and Japan begin to lose battles.

Churchill, Roosevelt, and Mackenzie King confer in Quebec.

DOUGLAS AND HIS TIMES	CANADA AND THE WORLD
1944	**1944**
Douglas resigns his federal seat to contest the Saskatchewan election on June 15; the CCF wins forty-seven out of fifty-two seats and establishes a "beachhead of socialism on a continent of capitalism"; Douglas is premier.	D-Day invasion by the Allies on June 6 begins the liberation of Europe.
	Vietnam declares independence from France.
Douglas government passes the Farm Security Act, which protects farmers from creditors; the federal government challenges it in the courts.	In Canada, in response to the CCF victory in Saskatchewan, Prime Minister King introduces family allowances; a conscription crisis again divides Canadians along French/English lines, but is less divisive than in World War I.
1945	**1945**
While visiting Canadian troops in Europe, Douglas re-injures his knee; it bothers him on and off for the rest of his life.	Germany surrenders on May 8; the U.S. drops atomic bombs on Japan on August 6 and 9; Japan surrenders on September 2.
At the federal-provincial conference, all premiers oppose Mackenzie King's plan for the postwar era except Douglas, who believes in strong central government.	United Nations Charter is signed on June 26; Canada is one of the signatories.
	Mackenzie King uses anti-CCF rhetoric to win the federal election; the CCF elects twenty-eight, including eighteen from Saskatchewan.
Douglas invites Japanese-Canadians to resettle in Saskatchewan.	Family allowances are introduced in Britain.
	1946
	Winston Churchill introduces the term "Iron Curtain" to describe the alienation between the Eastern Bloc and the West that is developing into the Cold War.

DOUGLAS AND HIS TIMES

CANADA AND THE WORLD

1947
CCF launches Saskatchewan-wide free hospital care.

1947
U.S. Congress passes the Taft-Hartley Act restricting the rights of labour unions.

1948
In the Saskatchewan election, the Liberals gain seats by charging that Douglas takes his orders from Moscow.

1948
Louis St. Laurent becomes the Liberal prime minister.

1949
Douglas government establishes the Saskatchewan Arts Board (the first in North America) and a provincial archive.

1949
Newfoundland joins Confederation; Canada joins the North Atlantic Treaty Organization (NATO); in the federal election, the CCF caucus drops to thirteen.

Communist Peoples' Republic of China is proclaimed.

The U.S.S.R. tests its first atom bomb.

1950
Since 1944, the Douglas government has established a small claims court (the first in North America), set a minimum wage and a forty-hour week, and doubled union membership.

1950
North Korea invades South Korea.

U.S. passes a law severely restricting communists.

1952
U.S. tests the first hydrogen bomb.

1953
In the federal election, the CCF wins twenty-three seats.

Korean armistice signed.

DOUGLAS AND HIS TIMES

CANADA AND THE WORLD

1954
Douglas government imposes wage restraints; power utility unions threaten a strike; back-to-work legislation is drawn up.

1954
On national television, U.S. Senator Joseph McCarthy searches for communists.

1956
Fifty per cent of Canadians are covered by voluntary private or nonprofit prepaid medical plans.

1957
Hospital Insurance and Diagnostic Act passed in Canada.

In June, John Diefenbaker's PC party defeats the Liberals; the CCF elects twenty-five.

U.S.S.R. launches Sputnik, the first earth satellite.

1958
Federal government approves a South Saskatchewan River dam, which the Douglas government has been asking for since 1944.

1958
In March, the Diefenbaker government wins 208 seats; having won only 8, the CCF intensifies efforts to make an alliance with labour.

1959
When travelling in Italy, Douglas gives a speech despite having developed Bell's palsy.

In April, Douglas announces decision to forge ahead with medicare.

1959
St. Lawrence Seaway opens.

Fidel Castro becomes the Premier of Cuba and soon allies himself with the U.S.S.R.

DOUGLAS AND HIS TIMES

1960
Medicare is the key issue in the June election in Saskatchewan; Douglas wins a solid majority, but the doctors continue to stall.

1961
In August, Douglas wins the national leadership of the newly formed New Democratic Party (NDP); he calls for a special session of the provincial legislature to enact medicare; in November, Douglas steps down as premier to be replaced by Woodrow Lloyd.

1962
In the June federal election, the campaign in Saskatchewan is ugly; Douglas is defeated in Regina; in a subsequent by-election, he wins a seat in Burnaby-Coquitlam in B.C.

On July 1, the start-up day for medicare, 90 per cent of Saskatchewan doctors strike; replacement doctors are brought in; the strike ends by the end of the month.

1963
In Ottawa, Douglas and the NDP hold the balance of power; like the CCF, the NDP serves as the conscience of Parliament and nudges the government toward medicare, pensions, and labour reforms.

CANADA AND THE WORLD

1960
CCF is dissolved.

John F. Kennedy becomes President of the U.S.

1961
All Canadian provinces have hospital plans.

Cuban exiles with U.S. backing attempt unsuccessful invasion of Cuba at the Bay of Pigs.

Berlin Wall separates East and West Germany.

1962
In Canada, Diefenbaker and the PC party sweep the west; no NDP candidates are elected in Saskatchewan.

U.S. establishes a military council in South Vietnam; the Cuban Missile Crisis brings the U.S.S.R. and the U.S. to the brink of war.

1963
Liberals under Lester Pearson form a minority government in Canada.

In the U.S., race riots and freedom marches inflame the country; the government sends troops into Vietnam; President Kennedy is assassinated.

DOUGLAS AND HIS TIMES

1964
The Liberals in Saskatchewan defeat the NDP government; in twenty years in power the NDP has eliminated the provincial debt.

1967
Gardiner Dam is opened on Diefenbaker Lake in Douglas Provincial Park.

1968
In a televised election debate between three party leaders, Douglas steals the show; the NDP wins twenty-two seats, but Douglas loses his; in July he wins a by-election in Nanaimo-Cowichan-The Islands.

CANADA AND THE WORLD

1965
Judge Emmett Hall presents his report on health services, which recommends medicare for all Canada; the Maple Leaf becomes Canada's flag.

American students demonstrate against the war in Vietnam.

1966
Medical Care Act passed in Canada.

1967
Canada celebrates 100 years of Confederation; France's President De Gaulle shouts *"Vive le Québec libre."*

1968
Pierre Trudeau replaces Pearson as leader of the Liberals and wins the federal election in Canada.

Martin Luther King and Robert Kennedy are assassinated in the U.S.

DOUGLAS AND HIS TIMES

1969
Douglas is critical of U.S. policy in Vietnam.

1970
In what is called "his finest hour, certainly his loneliest," Douglas and the NDP caucus protest the use of the War Measures Act; his stand causes sharp divisions in the NDP.

1971
Douglas is succeeded by David Lewis as the NDP leader; Douglas stays on as energy critic.

1972
Douglas punches a hold-up man in Jamaica.

1975
While speaking in the house, Douglas collapses with a bleeding ulcer.

CANADA AND THE WORLD

1969
NDP wins the Manitoba election; the Waffle faction of the party argues for a more socialist platform.

Neil Armstrong is the first man to walk on the moon.

1970
In Canada, Trudeau's government invokes the War Measures Act during the FLQ Crisis.

1971
NDP wins the Saskatchewan election; the Douglas-Coldwell Foundation, a left-wing think tank, is founded.

Canada and China exchange envoys and set the stage for western diplomatic recognition of China.

1972
All Canadian provinces have joined medicare.

NDP wins the B.C. election.

1975
Communists force U.S. troops out of Vietnam.

DOUGLAS AND HIS TIMES

1979
Douglas resigns his seat in Parliament; he becomes Chair of the Douglas-Coldwell Foundation; he leads a delegation to China.

1980
Douglas is made a Companion of the Order of Canada.

1981
Douglas is diagnosed with inoperable cancer.

1983
Although very sick, Douglas speaks at the NDP convention and fiftieth anniversary of the Regina Manifesto; he receives a half-hour standing ovation.

1984
Douglas is hit by a bus and is hospitalized for weeks.

1985
On December 5, Douglas receives the Saskatchewan Award of Merit; it is his final public appearance.

1986
Tommy Douglas dies on February 24.

CANADA AND THE WORLD

1980
Judge Hall says Canada's medicare system is one of the very best in the world.

Sources Consulted

Interview transcripts

THOMAS, Lewis H., ed., *The Making of a Socialist: The Recollections of T.C. Douglas*, Edmonton: University of Alberta Press, 1982.

Biographies

MCLEOD, Thomas H. and MCLEOD, Ian, *Tommy Douglas: The Road to Jerusalem*, Edmonton: Hurtig, 1987.

SHACKLETON, Doris French, *Tommy Douglas*, Toronto: McLelland & Stewart, 1975.

Political analysis

TYRE, Robert, *Douglas in Saskatchewan: The Story of a Socialist Experiment*, Vancouver: Mitchell Press, 1962.

Speeches

LOVICK, L.D., ed., *Till Power Is Brought to Pooling: Tommy Douglas Speaks*, Lantzville, B.C.: Oolichan, 1979.

Anecdotes

Whelan, Ed and Pemrose, *Touched by Tommy*, Regina: Whelan Publications, 1990.

Videos

Folks Call Me Tommy, produced by Don List, directed by Don List and Brock Stevens, Regina: Birdsong Films, 1982.

Tommy Douglas: Keeper of the Flame, written by Donald Brittain, produced and directed by Elise Swerhone, National Film Board, 1986.

Tommy Douglas: In His Own Words, produced and directed by Lief Storm, Regina: Pebble Beach Productions, in association with History Television and Saskatchewan Communications Network-SCN, 1998.

Index

Printed in June 2000
at Marc Veilleux Imprimeur Inc.,
Boucherville (Québec).